Designing Technology Training for Older Adults in Continuing Care Retirement Communities

Human Factors & Aging Series

Series Editors

Wendy A. Rogers and Arthur D. Fisk

School of Psychology

Georgia Institute of Technology – Atlanta, Georgia

Published Titles

Designing Technology Training for Older Adults in Continuing Care Retirement Communities

Shelia R. Cotten, Elizabeth A. Yost, Ronald W. Berkowsky, Vicki Winstead, and William A. Anderson

Designing Training and Instructional Programs for Older Adults

Sara J. Czaja and Joseph Sharit

Designing Telehealth for an Aging Population: A Human Factors Perspective

Neil Charness, George Demiris, and Elizabeth Krupinski

Designing Displays for Older Adults

Richard Pak and Anne McLaughlin

Designing for Older Adults: Principles and Creative Human Factors Approaches, Second Edition

Arthur D. Fisk, Wendy A. Rogers, Neil Charness, Sara J. Czaja, and Joseph Sharit

Human Factors
& Aging Series

Designing Technology Training for Older Adults in Continuing Care Retirement Communities

Shelia R. Cotten
Elizabeth A. Yost
Ronald W. Berkowsky
Vicki Winstead
William A. Anderson

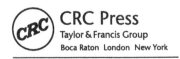

CRC Press
Taylor & Francis Group
Boca Raton London New York

CRC Press is an imprint of the
Taylor & Francis Group, an **informa** business

CRC Press
Taylor & Francis Group
6000 Broken Sound Parkway NW, Suite 300
Boca Raton, FL 33487-2742

Printed on acid-free paper
Version Date: 20161027

International Standard Book Number-13: 978-1-4987-1812-7 (Paperback)

Library of Congress Cataloging-in-Publication Data

Names: Cotten, Shelia R.
Title: Designing technology training for older adults in continuing care retirement communities / Shelia R. Cotten, Elizabeth A. Yost, Ronald W. Berkowsky, Vicki Winstead and William A. Anderson.
Description: Boca Raton, FL : CRC Press, 2017. | Includes bibliographical references and index.
Identifiers: LCCN 2016029415 | ISBN 9781498718127 (pbk.)
Subjects: LCSH: Computers and older people. | Internet and older people. | Retirement communities--Activity programs.
Classification: LCC QA76.9.O43 C67 2017 | DDC 004.084/6--dc23
LC record available at https://lccn.loc.gov/2016029415

Visit the Taylor & Francis Web site at
http://www.taylorandfrancis.com

and the CRC Press Web site at
http://www.crcpress.com

Printed and bound in the United States of America by
Edwards Brothers Malloy on sustainably sourced paper

We dedicate this book to all of the CCRC residents who participated in our study—many had never used a computer before, and they inspired us with their determination while making us laugh and filling our (work) days with joy. Without them, this book would not be possible.

Contents

Preface.. xiii
Acknowledgments xvii
Authors..xix

Chapter 1 Introduction and purpose 1
1.1   Importance of technology use for older adults in
        continuing care retirement communities.. 1
1.2   Aging population demographics 2
        1.2.1   Global trends 2
        1.2.2   U.S. trends.. 6
1.3   Value of technology for increasing quality of life for
        older adults 9
1.4   Technology use among older adults 9
1.5   Residential communities for older adults 11
1.6   Objectives for the book 12
Recommended readings.. 13
        Demographics of aging.. 13
        ICT use 14

**Chapter 2 Continuing care retirement communities and
                    the need for technology training** 15
2.1   The CCRC model 15
2.2   Historical development of CCRCs... 17
        2.2.1   Statistics on independent living communities
                    and assisted living communities.. 18
        2.2.2   Independent versus assisted living....................................... 18
        2.2.3   Care community analogues abroad....................................... 20
2.3   The stress of transition.. 22
        2.3.1   Adjusting to the transition 23
        2.3.2   The impacts on social interactions and relationships 25
2.4   Older adults and technology usage 26
        2.4.1   Barriers to usage among older adults in a CCRC.............. 28

      2.4.2   Technology use and connection to modern society 29
Recommended readings.. 31
    More about CCRCs.. 31
    Technology use among older adults 31

Chapter 3 A prototype study **33**
3.1   The idea for the study 33
3.2   Gaining entrance 34
3.3   Selecting the right context... 35
3.4   Preparation 36
      3.4.1   Assistive devices... 38
      3.4.2   Recruiting 40
3.5   Staging the intervention: where, when, and how to set up
      the training sessions.. 41
      3.5.1   Where: find lots of room....................................... 41
      3.5.2   When: scheduling and fitting into CCRC schedules.......... 44
      3.5.3   How: reducing distractions and frustrations—making
              it a good experience... 46
3.6   Implementation.. 47
3.7   Retention 49
3.8   Assessment 51
3.9   Lessons learned 52
Recommended readings.. 53

**Chapter 4 Complexities of and best practices for implementing
                 technology training in continuing care retirement
                 communities.. 55**
4.1   Understanding the learner 56
      4.1.1   Physical health and mobility of older learners.................. 57
      4.1.2   Dexterity and visual and hearing ability 58
      4.1.3   Cognitive ability 59
4.2   Organizing the environment.. 61
      4.2.1   Physical layout of the classroom........................... 61
      4.2.2   Scheduling: "You don't mess with bingo" 63
4.3   Ensuring the proper equipment... 64
4.4   Designing and presenting the content 67
      4.4.1   To lecture or not to lecture 68
      4.4.2   Taking the content home 68
4.5   Engaging and motivating participants.................................. 70
      4.5.1   Training the trainer 70
      4.5.2   The importance of a supportive teaching team 71
      4.5.3   Practice makes perfect 72

4.5.4   Ask your neighbor—promoting a community
         where residents help one another 73
4.6   Other considerations 75
       4.6.1   The importance of engaged activity directors 75
       4.6.2   Enabling the older adult to adapt to rapidly
                changing technology 76
       4.6.3   Expecting attrition 78
4.7   Summary of best practices 79
Recommended readings 82

Chapter 5   Value of technology training **83**
5.1   Changing attitudes and self-efficacy 84
       5.1.1   Attitudes toward ICTs 85
       5.1.2   Self-efficacy 88
5.2   Technology use across the study 90
5.3   Quality of life outcomes 94
       5.3.1   Depression and loneliness 94
       5.3.2   Psychological well-being 96
       5.3.3   Spatial and social barriers and connecting with others 97
       5.3.4   Case study—Ms. W.: Transcending spatial and
                social barriers 98
5.4   Tech training and understanding as a benefit unto itself 99
5.5   Conclusion 101
Recommended readings 101

**Chapter 6   Recruiting and retaining older adults in
             technology training programs** **103**
6.1   Recruitment 103
       6.1.1   Recruitment sessions 106
                6.1.1.1   Formal recruitment sessions 106
                6.1.1.2   Using family council or other
                           community meetings 109
                6.1.1.3   Informal recruitment sessions 109
       6.1.2   Special considerations for recruiting in
                research settings 110
       6.1.3   Recruiting at different care levels of the CCRC 112
6.2   Retention 113
       6.2.1   Needs 114
       6.2.2   Building rapport 115
       6.2.3   Class time 116
       6.2.4   Office hours 119
6.3   The role of the activity director in recruitment and retention 120

6.4   Role of incentives in recruitment and retention for research
       projects 121
6.5   Conclusion 122
Recommended readings.. 122

Chapter 7   Training decisions..**125**
7.1   Uniqueness of specific CCRC populations 125
7.2   Anticipated numbers... 127
7.3   Individual versus group training sessions 129
7.4   Training duration... 130
7.5   Training location.. 131
7.6   Who will do the training? 131
       7.6.1   Background and knowledge needed 132
       7.6.2   Interpersonal characteristics... 132
       7.6.3   Number of trainers and assistants needed 134
       7.6.4   Consistency in training personnel and methods............. 135
       7.6.5   Do it yourself or contract it out....................................... 135
       7.6.6   External contractor decisions—How to find and
                evaluate external trainers 136
7.7   Fit with CCRC population.. 140
Recommended readings.. 140

**Chapter 8   Current needs for technological access and use
                in continuing care retirement communities**..................... **141**
8.1   Interface..141
8.2   Access 143
8.3   Keep it simple.. 144
8.4   Continual support 144
8.5   The importance of outsiders for continued use 146
Recommended readings.. 147

**Chapter 9   The future of technology use among older adults
                in continuing care retirement communities**..................... **149**
9.1   Developments in the world of technology 149
9.2   What's for dinner? The inTRAnet in independent and
       assisted living communities 151
9.3   Virtual healthcare.. 154
       9.3.1   Healthcare via teleconferencing or videoconferencing....... 154
       9.3.2   Mobile health applications 155
9.4   Increased access and the importance of broadband 157
9.5   Changing interfaces 160
       9.5.1   The trouble with going from Windows
                Vista to Windows 8... 160

9.5.2 The move to mobile-friendly interfaces.............................. 163
9.6 Robotics and telepresence 164
9.7 The Internet of things 165
9.8 Conclusion 166
Recommended readings...167
Tablet usage among older adults...167
Technologies applicable for researchers and trainers to use in a CCRC setting..167

Chapter 10 Conclusions and final thoughts **169**
10.1 Thoughts on implementing training programs for older adults 169
10.2 Further considerations and reflections............................ 173

Bibliography.. 175
Appendix.. 181
Index 187

Preface

In an increasingly technological world, it has become substantially easier for individuals to manage their own healthcare. Through the use of a computer and the Internet, people can go online to gather information on their diagnosis, peruse potential treatment options, find doctors and healthcare centers that specialize in the treatment of illnesses, and even look up directions and routes on how to get to the doctors and healthcare centers, whether by driving or taking public transportation.

Now imagine that you have received a diagnosis for a new chronic condition and wish to receive the best of care; however, imagine now that you are an 80-year-old person living in an assisted living community...

...and now imagine that you have never used a computer before. What may have been easy for most can be difficult or nearly impossible for an older adult with little to no computer experience. Without technology knowledge and skills, older adults cannot gather information and communicate the same way as others can, which can be a huge issue in a technology-based reality.

The goal of this book is to help others understand the complexities and the best practices in training older adults in continuing care retirement communities (CCRCs) to use information and communication technologies (ICTs). Much of our experience comes from our 5-year longitudinal study on the impacts of ICTs on the quality of life of older adults in CCRCs. In this project, we trained several hundred older adults living in CCRCs in how to use ICTs. We learned a lot from going through this project, with much of it related to the intricacies of working in CCRCs, specifics of the older adult population in CCRCs, and the importance and specifics of tailoring training for this group.

In the United States, it is expected that more than 10,000 people will turn 65 years of age each day for the next 20 years. As people age, they often relocate to be closer to family or to receive more help with their daily tasks. CCRCs are gaining in popularity and are expected to continue to be communities of care for specific populations of older adults in the foreseeable future. When older adults relocate, they are removed from their social networks, which can include family, close friends, neighbors, and group members (such as through church membership or a recreational club or league). Although the older adults may still interact with people in their established networks, often the form of interaction changes, and they are met with increasing difficulty in maintaining these connections—connections that are vital for health and well-being. As this population grows, technology may be one avenue that can be used to help mitigate some of these negative effects.

Technology is an important tool that has been incorporated into nearly every facet of our daily lives. A majority of people in the United States own or at least have access to an Internet-connected computer or laptop and use these devices frequently. You would also be hard pressed to walk along a given street and not see at least a few people tinkering away on their smartphones, whether making a phone call, checking email, surfing the Web, or playing with an app. Being a part of the twenty-first century mandates that we are all proficient users of technology. It is not simply for our jobs; it is a way of life. However, older adults are less likely to use ICTs and may feel disenfranchised from a society in which technology is so important and so ingrained. Not using ICTs limits not only their contact with others but also access to resources, including information that may be vital to their healthcare and well-being. That puts the nonuser at a disadvantage in almost every aspect of life: social, financial, and educational. It also limits the nonuser's ability to fully participate in everyday life and enjoy the benefits that are associated with using ICTs.

This book describes best practices for conducting ICT training in CCRCs. Educating the current CCRC population on ICTs can help address many negative influences on quality of life. This is a targeted group for training and thus the classes and training procedures should be tailored to address older adult populations. Through this experience, we learned how to enable participants to overcome various social and spatial barriers that they encountered, how to address physical challenges that were unique to certain participants, and the value of constant reinforcement of their technology use. An ongoing challenge was tailoring the training to each group. There is no "one size fits all" for this training, although we present best practices that facilitate training and design. What works with one group may need to be tweaked with the next, and what works with one program one way probably will change with the next technology software or hardware update. Being cognizant of these issues will help those who seek to assist older adults in crossing the digital divide from nonuser to successful ICT user.

Throughout our experience, we learned a tremendous amount not only about pedagogical processes but also about the everyday lives of the older adults we were training. We learned about their fears of being left out of society, left behind in this technological age, and being limited in their ability to physically connect with people and places. Although many of these individuals will never use technology in the ways you or I do, their enjoyment through the process was palpable. It was more than learning how to open an email or search for information online; the experience was also about learning the lingo and belonging to the tech-grounded society of their children and grandchildren. They taught us something too: how to persevere as instructors, and that, as one participant remarked to us, "You can teach an old dog new tricks." One day we will all be "old dogs," faced with the daunting process of learning the newest technology. It is our hope we face this challenge with the grace and humor of many of our participants.

Acknowledgments

This book would not have been possible without funding from the National Institute on Aging to support our study. The views expressed in this book represent those of the authors and not necessarily those of the National Institute on Aging. We are also grateful to the 19 continuing care retirement communities (CCRCs) that we worked with during the study. We appreciate the cooperation of administrators and activities directors who were so willing to assist us by allowing us (mostly) unfettered access to the spaces where we conducted the training. This often required them to make other arrangements for resident social and recreational activities, meetings, and so forth. They helped us recruit and sometimes were a part of the training process. We also appreciate their encouraging words to us and the residents/participants. However, it was the hundreds of older adults who participated in the various components of our project that meant so much to our project. Their willingness to attend a training session even when they did not feel like it, and their diligence and perseverance throughout the training were truly inspiring to all of us. We gained so much from working with them. Regardless of the long-term impacts of our project, we saw changes in outlook and engagement among so many participants that helped us to know the value of the work that we were doing. We heard many variations of the following quotes!

> These four walls get tiresome sometimes…. [it's] not exactly lonesome, but when you stay in your room all the time…it gets boring…. [The computer training] kept my mind active, and my doctor says I needed that, so I got it, and…it really broadened my horizons….I think the computer has opened up my horizons (Ms. M., age 90).
>
> Now I feel part of the human race. [Learning to use the computer] gave me an opportunity to grow more…. There's more out there I need to know…[to] increase my level of life (Ms. M., age 85).

We also appreciate the connections that Dr. Richard Allman, former director of the University of Alabama at Birmingham Center for Aging, helped forge for us. With any project of this type, having someone who is well connected with the communities in which you wish to work is critical. We appreciate his help in connecting us with several CCRCs. We are also appreciative of Joshua Richman, Tom Houston, Eta Berner, and Karlene Ball, and the various consultants who were all involved in the initial refinement of the proposal that was funded by the National Institute on Aging.

During the course of the 5-year training programs, we had several research assistants who helped us with the trainings, interviews, coding, manuscript development, and related project activities. We thank all of the students, both past and present, for their work with us on the project and their contributions to ensure the success of the project.

Authors

Shelia R. Cotten is a professor in the Department of Media and Information at Michigan State University. She is also the director of the Sparrow/MSU Center for Innovation and Research, and the director of the Trifecta Initiative. Prior to joining Michigan State University in 2013, she was a professor in the Department of Sociology at the University of Alabama at Birmingham. She studies technology use across the life course, and the health, educational, and social impacts of that use. Her current work focuses on identifying the specific pathways by which ICT use benefits older adults, as well as developing new technology-focused interventions designed to enhance the quality of life for older adults. She is a past chair of the Communication and Information Technologies section of the American Sociological Association (CITASA). In 2016, she won the William F. Ogburn Career Achievement Award from the Communication, Information Technologies, and Media Sociology section of the American Sociological Association. She feels very fortunate to have worked with the coauthors on this book, who were all PhD students working with her when she was a faculty member at the University of Alabama at Birmingham. She is also very thankful to all the collaborators, students (past and present), and participants who helped to make this project a success.

Elizabeth A. Yost earned her PhD in medical sociology with a specialization in gerontology at the University of Alabama at Birmingham. She is an assistant professor of sociology at Washington College in Chestertown, MD, where she teaches courses in medical sociology and public health. Her research focuses on quality of life and well-being in older adult populations and the impact of technology on quality-of-life outcomes across the life course. She feels extremely fortunate to have worked with such excellent colleagues on such a fulfilling project over the past 8 years.

Ronald W. Berkowsky earned his PhD from the University of Alabama at Birmingham. He currently works as a postdoctoral associate at the University of Miami School of Medicine. Specifically, he provides assistance in data collection and analysis as well as works as a consultant for the Center on Aging, housed in the Department of Psychiatry and Behavioral Sciences. Most of his efforts are directed toward the Center for Research and Education on Aging and Technology Enhancement (CREATE), a multidisciplinary and collaborative center that examines technology impacts in old age, with projects conducted at the University of Miami, Florida State University, and the Georgia Institute of Technology. His research focuses on the physical, mental, and social impacts of technology in old age and how technology helps or influences health information-seeking. Projects he is currently involved in at the Center on Aging include the development and testing of an updated version of the personal reminder information and social management (PRISM) system, a software application designed as a part of CREATE for older adults to promote connectivity and information-seeking; the testing and assessment of an online suite of programs designed to teach aging adults to better perform technology-based tasks necessary for functional living (e.g., using an ATM, using a cellular phone to fill a prescription); and an examination of the decision-making processes of older adults in technology adoption and what factors (e.g., cognitive cost) affect this process. He feels very fortunate to have had the privilege of working with the coauthors on the research described in this book and is thankful to have worked with an amazing team of researchers and an engaged and exciting group of intervention participants.

Vicki Winstead earned her PhD from the University of Alabama at Birmingham. She currently works as a program manager for several projects that include developing and using strategies to recognize and manage care-resistant behaviors in residents with dementia in long-term care communities and examining the perceptions of caregivers as they interact with these residents during daily provision of care. She is responsible for coordinating and implementing several different interventions in long-term care communities that test the efficacy of these strategies during the provision of daily oral care. She also serves as a clinical data analyst for these projects. The goal of this research is to translate the findings into training for caregivers in long-term care. Her research focuses on the development of activities that mitigate the effects of the disease process in dementia for residents in various levels of long-term care communities. She specifically plans to develop resources for leisure activities for residents in assisted living with mild cognitive impairment that attenuate the effects of further cognitive decline by building cognitive reserve.

This, of course, will include technology! She worked closely with her coauthors on the project referenced in this book for 5 years and describes it as an "opportunity of a lifetime. The experience was enriching for trainer and trainee alike." She believes that spending the amount of time the project required with the wonderful participants of independent and assisted living communities also allowed a glimpse into their daily lives. She found that they met the challenges and limitations of growing older with courage and grace.

William A. Anderson is a research associate in the Division of Preventive Medicine in the School of Medicine at the University of Alabama at Birmingham (UAB). While finishing his PhD at UAB, he served as the project manager for the ICTs and Quality of Life study. After finishing his PhD, he spent time as a research study manager and qualitative researcher in the Division of Infectious Diseases in the UAB School of Medicine. In this role, he coordinated several local and national research studies looking at the factors associated with engagement and retention in care among people living with HIV/AIDS. In his current role in the Division of Preventive Medicine, he assists researchers within the division with grant proposal and manuscript preparation. His research interests include the system- and societal-level factors affecting healthcare and health inequalities. He fondly remembers his time working with older adults in CCRCs and his collaborators on the ICTs and Quality of Life study.

chapter one

Introduction and purpose

1.1 Importance of technology use for older adults in continuing care retirement communities

Ms. W. is an 87-year-old woman who lives in an assisted living community in Alabama. She has never been married, has no children, and only has one friend who lives several states away who she gets to see with any regularity. Other residents report that she rarely participates in group activities. She uses a wheelchair to transport herself. When we met Ms. W., she seemed lonely and somewhat depressed. She enrolled in our computer training program at the encouragement of the activities director. Over the course of training, Ms. W. became more outgoing and began to interact in other activities throughout the community. She also had a lot of fun—at one point, she mentioned that she had "gotten her hair done" twice a week for all her life, never missing an appointment, but during the training program she had forgotten about a hair appointment because she was so excited for "computer class!" At the end of the training program, Ms. W. said, "I'm a hot 87-year-old computer expert. I know how to Google!" She had even reconnected with a high school friend via email. Although not all older adults who learn to use computers and the Internet will respond like Ms. W., our research shows that older adults in continuing care retirement communities (CCRCs) can overcome the digital divide, reconnect with family and friends, and gain skills to enhance their quality of life.

We decided to write this book as we have seen the benefits for the quality of life that learning to use computers and the Internet can bestow on older adults in different types of care communities. There are no books available that focus on training older adults in CCRCs to use various types of technology. Although some older adults may find general technology use books beneficial as they try to learn to use computers or other technologies, such resources are frequently not sufficient; older adults often need tailored instruction and materials that cannot be found in "off the shelf" books. Older adults who move into these communities have special needs that necessitate different recruitment and training than what older adults in the general community require. The training methods provided in this book should be applicable to the general community of older adults too; however, the converse of this would not be true for the majority of CCRC residents.

There will be a rapid increase in the number of older adults in the next few decades (as detailed in the next section), accompanied by rapid changes in information and communication technologies (ICTs), and unprecedented growth in the number of independent and assisted living communities nationwide. Therefore, it is important to consider why older adults may want to use ICTs and how they could benefit from them as well as the best ways to help activity directors, caregivers, providers, and older adults keep up with changing technology. This information should make it easier for owners and administrators of CCRCs to decide whether they should offer training to their residents or whether using an outside organization to assist with this process would be more beneficial. Regardless of the approach taken, the material in this book serves as a best-practice guide for thinking about technology training for older adults in CCRCs. Given the increasing portion of the population moving into older demographic age groups, utilizing proven methods for keeping older adults connected and engaged will be critical for CCRC administrators and others who work with the growing population of older adults. The methods that we describe will likely be useful for teaching future cohorts of older adults to use novel technologies that perhaps are not available or have not even been created at this time.

The remainder of this chapter provides a comprehensive view of aging demographics, technology use among older adults, and the benefits of technology use in an aging population. Also detailed are the key audiences targeted in this book and what each can learn from this material.

1.2 Aging population demographics

1.2.1 Global trends

The aging population continues to grow globally. Estimates project that the global proportion of individuals over the age of 65 will double from 7.8% (524 million individuals) in 2010 to approximately 16.7% (1.5 billion individuals) in 2050. Figure 1.1 details the changes in percent population and population size of the worldwide older adult population from 2010 to 2050.

Growth of the older adult population is expected to continue as healthcare and technology continue to improve health outcomes and fertility rates continue to decline. This doubling of the proportion of the population over the age of 65 has profound implications for economic and social policy. Although the change in the aging population is occurring globally, rates differ greatly between developing and developed countries.

Developed countries—ones that have undergone demographic transitions and industrialization—have long been thought to be unduly burdened by this population shift. As individuals in these countries are living

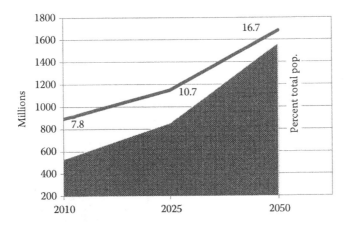

Figure 1.1 World population and the percentage of the total population aged 65 and older. Not only is the world population growing, but the percentage of older adults is also expected to grow. By 2050, 16.7% of the total population will be over the age of 65.

longer and children are considered more of an expense, fertility rates have dropped below replacement rates of 2.1 children per woman. This leads to a reduced workforce as older adults age out of the workforce and fewer children are born to replace them.

Countries throughout Europe and Asia are facing significant issues in workforce decline and shifting population pyramid structures. Other developed countries, such as the United States, Canada, and Australia, are experiencing slow growth in their workforce while still experiencing a growing population of people over the age of 65 who are often dependent on government welfare programs funded by taxes on working-age individuals. Population pyramids (Figure 1.2) detail the projected changing structure of the global population from 2010 to 2050.

With a reduced workforce and overall change in the number of aging individuals, some developed countries are confronting issues of increased numbers of individuals on social welfare programs in older age, and the need for greater resources for long-term care. As most developed countries are at or below the replacement rate—the number of children born per woman to keep the population rate stable—the overall population of many industrialized nations is declining. With fewer children being born and the population continuing to age, the issues of long-term care and social welfare programs will only become more significant as the next phase of demographic transition occurs.

Not only are the overall populations of these countries continuing to age, but the numbers of oldest old are continuing to increase as well.

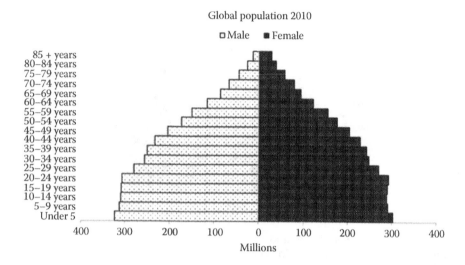

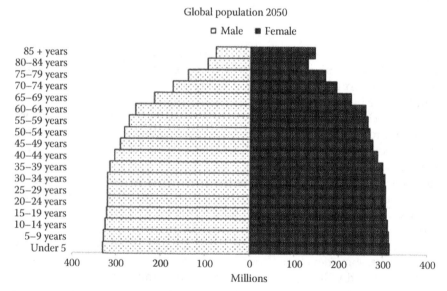

Figure 1.2 Global population pyramid for 2010 and 2050. By 2050 the shape of the global population pyramid is expected to shift from a traditional pyramid structure to a more column-like structure as the population grows older.

The oldest old—those 85 years of age and older—are often the portion of the older adult population that is most burdened by chronic disease. Although the numbers differ greatly between countries, the oldest old as a total portion of the global population is expected to increase 151%

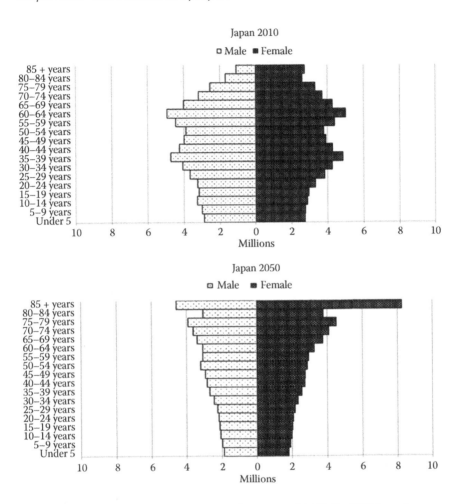

Figure 1.3 Population pyramid for Japan for 2010 and 2050. By 2050 Japan's population pyramid is expected to flip, with a majority of the population being over the age of 65.

between 2005 and 2030. Japan will be most impacted by this aging segment of the population. By 2050, 40% of Japan's population will be 65 or older, and Japan will have the greatest percentage of oldest old in the world. Figure 1.3 shows the projected growth and distribution by sex of Japan's older adult population from 2010 to 2050. The total portion of the oldest old will not increase quite as rapidly for the United States and some other newer developed countries.

Overall, developed countries are experiencing a significant demographic transition as the aging population continues to grow. Economic and social policies are being designed and implemented to address the changing population in developed countries, although they are not the only countries experiencing changes in their aging populations. Developing countries also have aging populations for which they are not structurally equipped. With increases in healthcare, individuals are living longer. In addition, many developing countries have experienced an epidemiological shift and are now dealing with chronic health issues more than acute health issues. As individuals are living longer, many developing countries are seeing a dramatic increase in life expectancy. Because of advances in healthcare, many developing countries are beginning to see increasing life expectancies and will soon be facing similar issues.

China is a unique and extreme example of aging in a developing country. Although China has made significant growth in the last three decades, it remains a developing country by the World Bank standards, as its per capita income is only a fraction of that of developed countries. The population of China is changing. Since the implementation of the one-child policy in China in 1979, the growth of China's population has been stunted. In 2000, 10.1% of China's population was over the age of 65. By 2050, it is projected to be 24% of the population, thus exceeding the global average.

1.2.2   U.S. trends

As the global population ages, the United States is also experiencing a graying of its adult population. This corresponds to the aging of the baby boomer population. Although the United States remains one of the youngest developed countries, compared to other developed countries, it has the greatest number of adults aged 65 and over and the greatest number of adults aged 85 and over. Among developed nations, the United States is second youngest to Russia in terms of median population age. Globally, the United States has the third-largest older adult population, with China having the first and India having the second.

The impact the aging baby boomers will have on U.S. demographics is significant. Baby boomers are individuals born between World War II and the mid-1960s. This "boom" represented a significant spike in fertility rates in the United States. As the first baby boomer turned 65 in 2011, this spike in the population is now resulting in a significant demographic shift in the United States. Figure 1.4 shows how the aging of the baby boomer generation will impact the structure of the population pyramids from 2010 to 2050. Because the United States is still a relatively young developed country, the demographics of the country including, but not limited to, the older adult population will continue to change. The

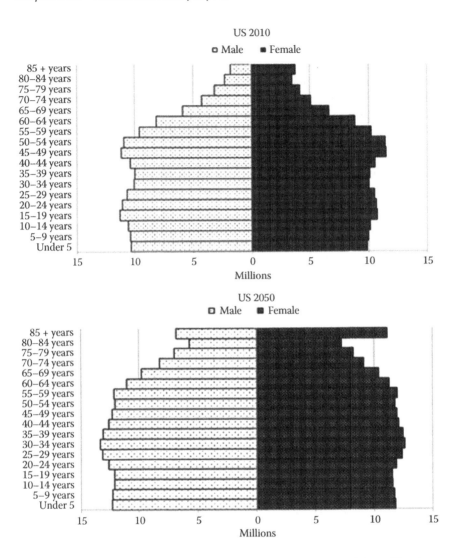

Figure 1.4 Population pyramid for the United States for 2010 and 2050. The shape of the population pyramid in the United States is set to change dramatically as the population ages. The pyramid shows the dramatic increase in adults 65 years of age and older in the United States by 2050.

median age, dependency ratios, sex, and race of the older adult population is expected to experience significant transition as the baby boomers continue to age. These changes impact the number of workers in an economy, the number of individuals able to participate in active military service, and the amount paid into and withdrawn from federal aging programs.

Although the United States experiences significant population growth from immigrants, the racial and ethnic composition of the older adult population should not be greatly impacted in the short term. As immigrants tend to be under 40 years of age, most will not be counted in the older adult population for at least another 25 years. However, by 2050, these demographics have the potential to shift dramatically, with almost 40% of the older adults in the United States reporting a minority racial status. Although the racial composition will vary between older adults and the oldest old, projections based on the 2010 Census suggest that the majority racial category among all older adults in 2050 will remain "white." However, all categories of racial minority groups are expected to increase, with the largest change being seen in Hispanic oldest old (85 years of age and older) populations.

Sex ratio is another characteristic expected to see dramatic changes in the immediate future. In 2012, there were 77.3 men for every 100 women over the age of 65. Over the age of 90, there were 40.3 men for every 100 women. By 2050, it is projected that there will be 81.5 men for every 100 women over the age of 65 and 52.7 men per 100 women over 90 years of age. Although women continue to have a longer life expectancy than their male counterparts, the gap is narrowing. Men are beginning to live longer, with the greatest change being in the sex ratios of the oldest old.

This shift in the sex ratios of the aging population has many interesting ramifications. As women tend to have longer life expectancies, they are more likely to live alone, rely on family members, and be widowed. As the percentage of men living longer increases, more women will retain their partners, and perhaps be able to age in place longer or rely on other family members less. This could also be a call for more CCRCs to have multiple options for couples who wish to continue living together.

As the population in the United States continues to age and grow, the country will face unique social and economic challenges. The well-being of this continuously aging population is of particular concern. As individuals live longer, they often reduce the number of working hours or retire, which limits their income; chronic illnesses develop, thus limiting their physical and psychological abilities. They also often relocate closer to family and perhaps further from friends, thus impacting their social, mental, and physical well-being. These changes are significant not only for individuals and families (e.g., caregiving and retirement planning), but also for society at large (e.g., social security programs, workforce factors, and long-term care options).

1.3 Value of technology for increasing quality of life for older adults

As compared to younger age groups, older adults often experience higher levels of loneliness, social isolation, depression, bereavement, health decline, and disabilities. When these co-occur, the quality of life for older adults can be even more compromised. Although a significant portion of older adults will experience one or more of these issues, recent research suggests that Internet activities can help to mitigate or negate the negative effects of these declines.

Research examining how technology use is related to various aspects of quality of life has increased in the past decade. One way in which Internet usage by older adults enhances well-being is that it enables them to maintain contact with their social networks, both strong and weak social ties. In doing this, they can exchange social support and gather information to help them make decisions, which all enhance well-being. Communicating with both strong and weak social ties is a main way through which Internet use is purported to affect well-being, through increasing social support, social contacts, and social connectedness.

Recent studies utilizing samples of older adults report that Internet use is associated with decreased depression, isolation, and loneliness, in addition to enhanced social support. Internet use can also help older adults and others with mobility and activity limitations. In this respect, using the Internet for interpersonal communication, as well as overcoming social and spatial boundaries, may be particularly salient for enhancing well-being.

Although this body of research illustrates the potential positive impacts of technology use for older adults, individuals must be users of the technologies in order to gain the benefits of them. The next section discusses the rates of technology use among older adults in the United States and how this compares to other age groups.

1.4 Technology use among older adults

The Pew Internet and American Life Study recently reported that although 86% of adults use the Internet, only 59% of adults aged 65 and over go online. The American Community Survey reported a similar number, with 65% of older adult households (65 years of age and older) having some sort of computer and 58% having access to the Internet. Older adults are a large portion of individuals in the United States who are not online, as shown in Figure 1.5.

Researchers have referred to this gap in use as the "digital divide." The initial term was used to describe the difference between users and

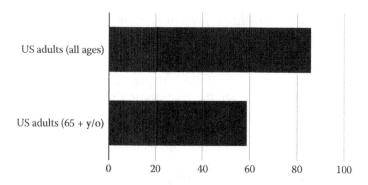

Figure 1.5 Internet use in the United States. Compared to adults of all ages in the United States, adults over 65 years of age are less likely to use the Internet.

nonusers. As more and more people are utilizing the Internet, the term "second-level digital divide" has been coined to describe the difference in use patterns and abilities to navigate technology. For older adults to be able to get the most out of their technology experience, access is not the only factor; they must also be given instruction on how to navigate the technology.

Older adults in the United States have different usage and adoption patterns, even within their demographic group. Among older adults online, there is a gap in use and in type of device they use to access the Internet. Among different age groups of adults, Internet use declines significantly among those older than 75. Although 74% of those 65–69 years old go online, only 47% of those 75–79 years old and 37% of those 80+ years old report that they go online. Also, the higher the income, the more likely the older adult is to report going online. Among those in the highest income bracket ($75,000+ annual household income), 90% report going online. Education also plays a role in adoption of technology. Older adults with higher levels of education are more likely to go online than those with lower levels of education. Older adults with high annual household incomes and higher levels of education, and who are between the ages of 65 and 74 are the most likely to be online. In terms of type of device, individuals 65 years and older report using desktops, laptops, and handheld computers less often than all younger age groups. Of individuals aged 65 and older, only 32% report using a handheld type of device to access the Internet, compared to 83% of people aged 15–34 years old. Aside from type of device, there is also a difference in Internet connection type between older and younger adults. The American Community Survey found that adults of age 65+ were the most likely age group to have dial-up access, and the least likely to have fiber-optic or mobile broadband connections.

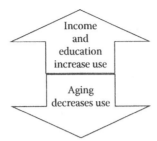

Figure 1.6 Factors that influence ICT use among older adults. Higher levels of income and education increase the likeliness of ICT use among older adult populations. Aging decreases ICT use among older adults.

Figure 1.6 summarizes the key factors that influence ICT use among older adults.

Although the number of older adults online continues to increase, older adults not only use different technologies but also use those technologies in different ways than their younger counterparts. Even among different generations of older adults online, there is a gap in type of technology and type of use. The younger old, those 65–84 years old, are more likely to be broadband adopters than the oldest old (85+ years of age). Older adults also report less smartphone, tablet, and other ICT adoption than younger cohorts. Although older adults are using different technologies, and using the technologies at different rates, research shows there are significant positive outcomes from technology use.

1.5   Residential communities for older adults

CCRCs, independent living communities (ILCs), and assisted living communities (ALCs) are uniquely designed communities for older adults. CCRCs contain a variety of options for residents. Often residents relocate to these communities to live out the rest of their lives. These types of communities incorporate all levels of care from independent homes to full-time skilled nursing options. ILCs are communities that only offer independent living arrangements. This can include homes to apartments that share common community spaces and activities. ALCs are communities designed to assist residents with some activities of daily living and instrumental activities of daily living. Most states mandate certain cognitive functions be met by residents to live in these communities. When residents no longer meet minimum cognitive requirements, they are required to move to communities that offer additional care options. All of these types of communities are expected to grow in the coming decades as the population ages.

To date, the largest study of the impact of technology on older adults in senior housing communities is the University of Alabama–Birmingham Information and Communication Technology Quality of Life Study. We carried out a 5-year longitudinal study on the impact of ICTs on the quality of life among older adults in CCRCs, specifically ILCs and ALCs. We found that ICT use was associated with decreased loneliness and depression, participants feeling more connected to friends and family, participants feeling less bothered by not seeing enough people close to them, and decreased social and spatial barriers.

Little other research has focused on older adults and technology in these types of communities. The majority of other research evaluating the impact of ICTs on older adults in CCRCs evaluates ICTs as assistive devices for maintaining independence, not technologies that help promote social well-being. A few small-scale studies have been conducted in different types of aging communities. Waldron, Gitelson, and Kelley (2005) evaluated how mediated communication (via email) impacted perceived social support among individuals who relocated to a retirement community.

1.6   Objectives for the book

We see the readership for this book falling into three broad categories:

1. Owners, CEOs, administrators, and activity directors of CCRCs and outreach organizations that work with older adults.
   For this group of readers, this book offers key insights into challenges that may need to be addressed when deciding whether to offer training in their communities or to older adults in other communal settings. It also provides the latest statistics on the percentages of older adults who use specific types of technologies as well as findings from research that examines the impacts of technology usage on older adults.
2. People working in organizations that specialize in designing technologies for universal access; people who design or target new technologies or instructional materials and programs for older adults; and people working through a variety of organizations (e.g., Connected Living, OasisNet, SeniorNet, Generations On Line, and so on) to help get older adults online.
   These readers will become aware of challenges related to conducting and disseminating technology training programs within CCRCs. They will also become more knowledgeable about physical and cognitive challenges facing older adults who move into these communities.

3. Educators and researchers, including human–computer interaction researchers and designers, gerontologists, sociologists, psychologists, media and communication researchers and systems developers, and human factors and ergonomics researchers and designers.

Readers in this group will learn about the largest study to date in the United States that addresses training older adults in CCRCs to use computers and the Internet. They will also gain information on the latest research findings from studies of this type, as well as best practices for designing technology interventions and training programs for residents of CCRCs.

This book offers all readers an in-depth view of what ICT training can offer older adults. It provides readers the knowledge, lessons learned, and helpful guidelines for implementing ICT research and use programs in CCRCs. Chapter 2 evaluates the history of CCRCs, and the possibilities that ICT training can bring to CCRC residents. Chapter 3 focuses on early considerations for conducting ICT research in CCRCs, including best practices for recruitment and retention. Chapter 4 includes complexities and best practices of implementing ICT training as well as the road blocks that might be experienced during training sessions. Chapter 5 describes the expected outcomes of ICT training for older adults with an analysis of past research. Chapter 6 identifies best practices for motivating older adults in CCRCs to best utilize the technology. Chapter 7 poses possible considerations for conducting training in CCRCs. Chapter 8 evaluates where technology is and some possible considerations it should take to assist older adult users. Chapter 9 provides future directions and evaluates the possibility of emerging technologies. Chapter 10 concludes the book, wrapping up the lessons learned and providing an argument for the relevance of emerging technologies. As the older adult population continues to age, addressing issues of well-being and connectedness is vital in maintaining a healthy and independent population.

Recommended readings

Demographics of aging

Dobriansky, P. J., Suzman, R. M., and Hodes, R. J. 2007. *Why population aging matters: A global perspective* (Publication 07–6134). Washington, DC: National Institute on Aging, National Institutes of Health, U.S. Department of Health and Human Services, U.S. Department of State.

Ortmann, J., Velkoff, V., and Hogan, H. 2014. *An aging nation: The older population in the United States* (Current Population Reports P25-1140). Washington, DC: U.S. Census Bureau.

Suzman, R. and Beard, J. 2011. *Global health and aging* (NIH Publication No. 11-7737). Washington, DC: National Institutes of Health and World Health Organization.

United Nations, Department of Economic and Social Affairs, Population Division. 2013. *World Population Ageing 2013* (ST/ESA/SER.A/348). Retrieved from http://www.un.org/en/development/desa/population/publications/pdf/ageing/WorldPopulationAgeing2013.pdf

ICT use

Berkowsky, R., Cotten, S. R., Yost, E., and Winstead, V. 2013. Attitudes towards and limitations to ICT use in assisted and independent living communities: Findings from a specially-designed technological intervention. *Educational Gerontology, 39*(11), 797–811.

Cotten, S. R., Anderson, W. A., and McCullough, B. M. 2013. Impact of Internet use on loneliness and contact with others among older adults: Cross-sectional analysis. *Journal of Medical Internet Research, 15*(2), e39. doi: 10.2196/jmir.2306.

Davison, E. and Cotten, S. R. 2010. Connection disparities: The importance of broadband connections in understanding today's digital divide. In E. Ferro, Y. Dwivedi, J. Gil-Garcia, and M. D. Williams (Eds.), *Overcoming digital divides: Constructing an equitable and competitive information society* (pp. 346–358). Hershey, Pennsylvania: IGI Global.

Sixsmith, A. and Gutman, G. 2013. *Technologies for active aging.* New York: Springer.

Smith, A. *Older adults and technology use.* Washington, DC: Pew Research Center. Retrieved from http://www.pewinternet.org/2014/04/03/older-adults-and-technology-use/

Winstead, V., Anderson, W. A., Yost, E., Cotten, S. R., Berkowsky, R., and Warr, A. 2013. You can teach an old dog new tricks: A qualitative analysis of how residents of senior living communities may use the web to overcome spatial and social barriers. *Journal of Applied Gerontology, 32*(5), 540–560.

Zheng, R. Z., Hill, R. D., and Gardner, M. K. 2013. *Engaging older adults with modern technology: Internet use and information access needs.* Hershey, Pennsylvania: IGI Global.

chapter two

Continuing care retirement communities and the need for technology training

2.1 The CCRC model

As baby boomers have come of retirement age, adequate senior housing has become important as an industry to meet the needs of an increasingly larger aging population. As illustrated in the demographic data in Chapter 1, the number of Americans aged 65 and older has dramatically increased and will continue to increase so that by the year 2050, the number of Americans aged 65 and older will comprise more than 20% of the US population, and many of them will prefer or require some level of a CCRC.

As baby boomers reach the age of those considered the oldest old (aged 85 and over), the necessity of long-term care will become even more essential. Chronic conditions or disease can necessitate greater levels of caregiving and limit an older adult's ability to remain in his or her own home. Significant out-of-pocket healthcare expenditures hinder access to care and quality of life and leave insufficient resources for other necessities. As a result, in the past few years, there has been a shift away from skilled nursing facilities toward a private market-based system, such as a CCRC.

A CCRC is a tiered senior housing model for older adults who can no longer maintain a private residence, need assistance with activities of daily living (ADLs), or require skilled nursing care. They offer older adults the opportunity to live at one location for the remainder of their lives, with options to receive greater assistance with care as their needs increase. CCRCs offer levels of care beginning with garden homes or apartment/condominiums where healthy older adults can live independently, but have access to services if needed. When assistance with everyday activities becomes necessary, they can move into assisted living or skilled nursing care facilities without leaving their retirement community. Memory care units are fast becoming a standard feature for CCRCs. The tiered levels are often referenced as a "continuum of care." This allows residents to age in place, thereby taking the stress of further relocation off of them and their potential caregivers, such as children or close relatives.

However, peace of mind for the future can be very expensive; the cost of moving into a CCRC is greater than other options for long-term care because residents are paying for the potential of future services as well as present services. Monthly charges can range up to $5000 per month, based on factors such as location and amenities, services provided by the CCRC, level of assistance, and choice of housing. However, the initial fee that guarantees access to care for the remainder of life can vary quite dramatically, ranging from over $100,000 up to $1,000,000. Due to consumer demand, many CCRCs are now offering older adults greater financing options with refunds available if certain conditions are met.

According to the AARP (2015), there are three types of contracts for residents:

1. *Life care contract.* This is the costliest option but guarantees unlimited care for life in the assisted living or skilled nursing options if needed.
2. *Modified contract.* This option offers needed services at a fixed rate over a set period of time. At the end of this time, the services are still available but at a higher rate.
3. *Fee-for-service contract.* This option may lower the initial entrance fee but assisted living and skilled nursing charges are assessed at the current rate.

CCRCs may vary in scope, size, and amenities, but three basic aspects are present in virtually every CCRC in the United States:

- All levels of care from independent living through skilled nursing are offered, with access available for life.
- Programs and amenities are available that contribute to healthier living with an emphasis on wellness. These can include state-of-the-art facilities, exercise programs, educational opportunities, travel opportunities, and appealing dining choices.
- Options for rest-of-life care in one place are available, based on the type of contract entered into.

The CCRC has continued its evolution with the "CCRC without walls." The concept of a CCRC without walls takes the types of services provided at a CCRC and makes them applicable to an in-home setting. As with a traditional CCRC, an entrance fee is required, as well as regular monthly fees and fees that apply to whatever services are offered in the package by the individual CCRC. This modern version of the CCRC is attractive to older adults because of its lower entrance fee for those who lack the financial resources to move into a traditional CCRC, allowing them to benefit from the services offered and the prospect of future care. However, the conditions for admission include stricter guidelines in terms of health, age, and number and type of chronic conditions. Another criterion is the necessity of a Medicare supplement insurance policy. Overall, initial admission into the CCRC is typically granted to healthy, independent older adults.

2.2   Historical development of CCRCs

Societal responsibility in caring for those in older ages of life is not a new or newly innovative concept. In fact, there is literary evidence of early homes or institutions for older, infirm adults as early as the late 1400s. Gabrielle Zerbia, a fifteenth century "gerontologist," authored a work, *Gerontocomia,* which was used as a handbook for institutionalized care for older adults who were sick or disabled. It included instructions for building design, staffing, and running the day-to day operations in the institution. Unfortunately, only males were considered worthy of this service.

The CCRC itself is not a new model; various forms of the modern CCRC have existed for many years. Many of the modern CCRCs still in operation today were founded more than 100 years ago. Institutions that predated the CCRC were originally built to care for those who could not care for themselves. Early institutions of care for older adults who had neither resources nor families who could offer support were called poorhouses, poor farms, or almshouses, and were prevalent in the eighteenth and nineteenth centuries. In the early twentieth century, very few older adults had sufficient resources to be able to afford a room in "senior" housing, such as a boarding house or convalescent home. Thus, alliances were formed between social institutions that included various religious and secular groups to provide what was then called an "old age home." The development of the old age home was an attempt to remove the stigma associated with names such as poorhouse or almshouse for older adults who were disabled or had chronic diseases. They would often require a resident to sign over their monetary and physical assets as a trade for care for the rest of their life, including nursing care, as they physically declined.

Similar to today's version, they were often called life care communities, referencing the nature of the service. As the model has evolved, similar groups remain the sponsors of many of the moderns CCRCs. Only about 18% of modern CCRCs are owned for profit, with most sponsored by not-for-profit entities. According to Zarem (2010) at LeadingAge Zeigler 100, a research organization for senior housing, some present-day CCRCs were begun as nursing homes, with other levels of care added over the years. CCRCs that were originally designed *as* a CCRC are designated as "purpose built," with all levels of care included as part of the design. Since the 1960s, CCRCs have increased in both number and the number of services they offer. Growth increased during the 1970s and 1980s as potential residents were attracted to choices in contracts. Between 10 and 20 purpose-built communities were constructed per year from around 1990 through the 2000s. CCRCs may be a single-campus organization or part of a system, with most of them being part of a system. The average CCRC has fewer than 300 units, with the largest having over 500 units.

2.2.1 Statistics on independent living communities and assisted living communities

The number of CCRCs being built continues to expand as the population ages. Table 2.1 gives the number of CCRCs and the distribution of independent living communities (ILCs) and assisted living communities (ALCs) as of 2014.

Of the CCRCs, 52% are faith-based, with only about 2% described as fraternal organizations. Some states regulate CCRCs, although the focus of oversight in states with explicit regulations is concentrated primarily on the financial aspects rather than the protection of consumers/residents. Most states regulate assisted living and skilled nursing levels of care. Interestingly, Ohio, with the second-highest number of CCRCs (150), has no state regulation of CCRCs.

2.2.2 Independent versus assisted living

Both independent living and assisted living levels of care are part of the CCRC model. However, there are communities in the United States that solely offer independent living, whereas others offer only assisted living. Some communities offer a combination of the two levels. The primary difference between assisted living and independent living is the level of care provided. Neither ALCs nor ILCs offer the 24/7 skilled nursing that is provided in nursing homes.

Table 2.1 Number of communities by type

	Communities	Units	Nonprofit (%)	For profit (%)
CCRC	1,900	676,000	81	19
ILC	1,500	179,000	2.3	97
ALC	22,000	851,400	22	78

Source: LeadingAge Ziegler 150. 2014. Retrieved from https://www.leadingage.org/uploadedFiles/Content/Members/Member_Services/LZ_100/LZ150-2014.pdf.

An ILC is senior housing that provides a safe and secure living environment but does not provide assistance with ADLs or medication assistance. Independent senior living residents are primarily able to live on their own with the option of limited assistance (provided by third-party home healthcare providers, if needed) and without around-the-clock supervision. However, other amenities are offered or provided, such as recreational and educational activities, dining services, light housekeeping, transportation, exercise programs, emergency alert systems, and onsite hair salons. They may be a part of the total package or may require separate fees to be used. An ILC is less costly than other levels of care and is appealing to older adults who are less able or willing to care for a home. Housing options can range from onsite garden homes that residents can rent or purchase, stand-alone senior apartments, and large senior-living complexes that have designated sections for independent living residents. ILCs are largely unregulated so that residents do not have to meet state-mandated physical or mental health criteria, except those required by the individual community or corporation that owns the community.

An ALC is designed to provide residents with assistance with daily activities such as medication, eating, bathing, dressing, and toileting. It was conceived as an alternative to nursing homes for residents who need assistance but do not require constant medical care, as is typical in skilled nursing facilities. In contrast to nursing homes, ALCs were intended to look like homes rather than clinical settings. They were designed as a resident-focused model that allowed the resident to preserve their autonomy, independence, and dignity while still being cared for. The terminology used to describe attributes of the assisted living community helped to sustain the perception of not being in a medical facility. The individuals are residents rather than patients, with their living quarters described as apartments rather than rooms. Use of the term "community" in contrast to "facility" helped to make the resident feel less institutionalized during the relocation process into continuing care.

In the development of the assisted living model, medical, physical, and psychosocial needs of the residents were treated as equal considerations. The development of the assisted living model was centered around the necessity of each resident maintaining dignity, privacy, and autonomy. Ensuring a resident-centered design for each of these attributes allows residents to maintain a perception of independence, in contrast to nursing homes in which these components become secondary to the medical needs of residents and more of a "staff-centered" environment. Table 2.2 details the percentage of residents in ALCs that need assistance with various activities of daily living (ADLs) and instrumental activities of daily living (IADLs).

Table 2.2 Most common ADLs and IADLS for residents in ALCs

Activities	Percentage of residents in ALCs needing assistance
Meal preparation	87
Medication management assistance	81
Bathing	64
Dressing	39
Toileting assistance	26
Transferring	19
Eating	12

Source: Assisted Living Federation of America. 2013. *What is assisted living?* Retrieved June 15, 2013, from http://www.alfa.org/alfa/Assisted_Living_Information.asp.

2.2.3   Care community analogues abroad

Globally, other nations are facing the same demographic challenges of caring for a growing population of older adults, including the challenges of providing care communities. As of 2012, 17.4% of people living in European nations in the European Union (EU) were aged 65 and older. This is expected to increase to 28% by 2020 due in part to a lower birth rate and a higher life expectancy. There is an emphasis on collaboration and partnerships between member states of the EU in addressing issues of housing and care for the increasing older adult population, especially those who have chronic conditions and need assistance, and in facilitating conditions for healthy independent aging. Various states have unique approaches to the challenges of caring for their oldest citizens.

In the Netherlands, responsibility for senior housing and welfare falls on local governments. The Dutch were innovators in the development of care institutions for older adults guided by the philosophy of "sheltered housing," a name for what they describe as "living in a protected environment." The Dutch model is described as "at least ten barrier-free flats with a care and support unit within a maximum distance of 250 meters. The housing units have a maximum size of two to three rooms between 55 and 70 square meters" (Stula, 2012).

Future plans include abolishing the necessity of skilled nursing facilities in favor of this model, with 85% of the cost paid through the social insurance system and the remaining cost paid by the individual resident.

Finland and Denmark have similar policies, with both countries emphasizing older adults remaining in their homes as long as possible with assistance from the social insurance system. In Finland, public assistance is available to adapt private homes with whatever is necessary to create a safe environment for older adult residents. This allows them to remain at home and retain independence as long as possible. For those requiring more care, there is an "intensive assisted living" option provided and funded by local governances, the welfare system, and private individuals. This has replaced the nursing home in Finland.

In the United Kingdom, the provision of "sheltered housing" for older adults has been systemically institutionalized throughout the country since the 1960s. The model is similar to the American CCRC, with a multi-level system based on the level of care required by the resident. Sheltered housing for healthier residents consists of individual apartments, which are designed and constructed to be a safe living environment and may include an emergency alert system and assistance with household chores. Care providers offer assistance, with up to nine care providers per 100 residents. "Very sheltered housing" is comparable to the ALC in the United States and offers a level of care in between independent living and a nursing home.

Care and housing for older adults is provided by private entities, local governments, or housing associations, and through charitable organizations (Stula, 2012). France has historically looked to the family as the primary provider of care for seniors in the home setting. Current models still emphasize at-home care but with the assistance of the state, social insurance, and the family. Respite care and adult day care, along with meal and care assistance provided by various charitable organizations, are helpful in enabling the older adult to remain at home. Future goals include allowing the citizens a choice between at-home care and a nursing home.

In less-developed countries such as India, older adults have fewer choices for care and housing. Both private and public homes are available, with residents reporting a large difference in the level of care between the two. There is little to no regulation for these homes, and people without resources or family to care for them must live in public homes for older adults.

In China, the majority of Chinese older adults live independently of family members, although the official stance of policymakers is that the care of older adults should be handled by the family without assistance from the state. This disconnection between policy and reality has led to a lack of adequate housing and care for older adults and especially those who are disabled or who need assistance.

As is clear from this discussion, the United States and countries abroad all face challenges with regard to caring for older adults with differing needs in different types of communities. Though the types of communities may vary somewhat, many of the challenges remain the same. For many older adults, the stress of transitioning into some type of care community can be highly salient. The next segment discusses in greater detail the stress of this transition for individuals moving into CCRCs.

2.3 The stress of transition

The transition into some form or level of a CCRC is a significant life event for older adults and can require considerable effort in adapting to the move. Many older adults prefer to continue living in their homes, also known as "aging in place." The decision to transition into a CCRC may be a result of declining physical and mental health, death of a spouse, or social concerns. However, the relocation may be necessitated because of a medical or personal crisis that leaves an older adult unable to continue living in his or her home. Older adults may decide to enter a continuing care community because of the advice or insistence of family members, such as adult children, nieces and nephews, or younger siblings, or their physician or other healthcare professional who may have observed mental or physical decline. In some cases, older adults may feel that they have no voice in the decision process, which can make the transition difficult.

The move into a CCRC can positively affect both physical and mental health because most care communities place an emphasis on meeting the needs of the whole person: social, emotional, and physical. This is especially true of the assisted living level, which offers physical assistance as well as social and emotional assistance. Residents who were previously socially isolated in their homes due to illness, loss of a spouse, distance from family, or loss of driving may be able to create new relationships within their CCRC.

Moving into a continuing care community has been associated with improved health and overall well-being because of increased opportunities for social contact, opportunities for participation in various activities, and assistance with ADLs for those who need the support. Although the move into a CCRC can have many positive outcomes on health and cognitive functioning, there are losses that come with the transitions as well.

The move may take older adults away from neighborhoods, social and religious institutions, and their friends and family. Many older adults have had to give up their cars and must depend on family members or friends for transportation, for social visits, or to attend church or other activities they enjoyed in the past. Therefore, much or all of their day may be spent within the CCRC itself.

They may experience feelings of isolation and loneliness, thereby affecting their physical and mental health. Reasons for the transition may be due to chronic health problems or the result of some type of crisis, which can include a physical health challenge, the death of a spouse, or some type of change in financial resources. Often they are left dealing with both the stress of the transition and the aftermath of the crisis. The move into a CCRC can put significant geographical distance between residents and their social networks, especially if the move is to another city or state. Fewer opportunities for contact and interaction result in less support, negatively impacting relationships. These "spatial barriers" restrict the ability of residents to actively participate beyond the four walls of the CCRC, especially for residents who require a higher level of care. For these residents, the bulk of their social life takes place within the community in which they reside. Activities offered in their particular community may or may not reflect their interests. Activity programs at CCRCs may contain activities that are considered low-cost, safe for residents, and easy to implement, with little or no input from residents.

Levels of physical activity may be affected when older adults are unable to continue previous social relationships that encouraged or facilitated physical activity. There can be deleterious effects on health when physical activity and participation in the types of activities that require some level of physical activity is decreased as a result of distance from previous social networks, such as moving into a CCRC.

2.3.1   *Adjusting to the transition*

Beyond the physical move, the adjustment period to a new residence can be stressful, affecting residents socially and physically. Perceptions of quality of life are higher for older adults when they have the option to continue living in their homes as compared to older adults who move into a CCRC.

The adjustment begins before the actual move, as older adults must find a place that fits their needed level of care, preferences, and budget. Relocation can be challenging when it requires older adults to leave their home, in essence physically separating individuals from their homes and communities and breaking their attachment to place. Hays (2002) described this attachment to place in terms of life narratives and the symbols (possessions) that accompany (and represent) the narrative. He further described it as a process that "creates linkages that tie an individual to a place." These links are important to the process of positive aging because the individual is imbued with a continuance of a lifelong trajectory of self-reliance and self-sufficiency.

The adjustment also includes the process of residents' decision-making about what to move with them and what to do with the rest of their possessions. As possessions often have symbolic value, this can become a painful process. Most of the time, the transition is to a smaller living space and thus physical possessions that are moved consist of only the necessary furniture or possessions that will fit into the smaller living space. This requires residents not only to choose what they need for daily living, but also choose the possessions that reflect a lifetime of who they are: possessions that symbolize their life.

Feelings of loss related to reduction or dissemination of personal possessions may be related to the symbolic value of the possessions rather than the actual physical loss. Physical possessions can represent meanings that individuals internalize as a form of self-validation and continuance of identity. Thus, making a choice to leave places and possessions that are symbols of identity can also negatively affect the well-being of residents. The loss of physical possessions may include the perception of losing previous life roles and former ways of life. Interviews with assisted living residents showed that some residents were bothered by the size of their new living space because, as one resident described, it does not allow for "adequate room for the past." Another resident explained how he stored possessions in his car that symbolized his life experiences because there was no place else to put them.

For many residents, the option to return home if the circumstances in a CCRC do not meet expectations is not available. Lack of financial resources and the cost of the move may dictate that their home must be sold. This leaves no option to "go home" if circumstances do not work out. The home can epitomize a lifetime of accumulation of possessions, the symbolic representation of a lifetime of memories; having to sell the family home can result in residents feeling insecure or that they have little or no control.

Relocation into a CCRC can interrupt the connections that represent a resident's lifetime. The challenges of transitioning and adapting to some form of continuing care can result in feelings of depression, isolation, and loneliness, in addition to experiencing the other types of losses discussed earlier, including loss of health and physical mobility, networks of friends, and possessions.

Residents may experience a disruption of patterns of daily living. Romero et al. (2010, p. 486) succinctly described the challenges that CCRCs face in how they design a community that addresses "the highly individualized and dynamic nature of quality of life"; older adults are not a homogeneous group and therefore what constitutes independence and autonomy for one individual does not fit another. Although Kane (2001) described life in a CCRC as a "synchronicity of normal life and ancillary services," residents often feel a line of delineation separating their previous life and their present life. Designing a model that addresses quality of life for older adults in communal living may be a difficult endeavor.

Residents of CCRCs must adjust to a daily routine as part of their care in their new community. This is especially true for residents of ALCs. Changes in their daily schedule and patterns may include alterations in both when and what they eat, how they take prescribed medications, transportation options, and availability for medical appointments, shopping, and errands, and social activities. Individuals in this setting may feel a loss of control over decisions and that they are "at the mercy" of the ALC administration.

Often, older adults have little control over the decision to move into a CCRC, with choices sometimes being made for them by others. Although any kind of relocation can be stressful for an older adult, the move into an assisted living community results in greater levels of stress and anxiety when compared to a move into an independent living community. This is especially the case when the move is involuntary because residents feel little or no control over the decision to move.

2.3.2 The impacts on social interactions and relationships

Social interactions and participation in activities offered in a CCRC can have a positive effect on cognition and promote feelings of well-being. However, for many older adults, the move into a CCRC gives them a perception of compression of their social life because of illness or distance or a combination of the two. Winstead et al. (2013, p. 541) defined social compression as social barriers that "represent the negative qualitative changes in social interactions and social ties." Older adults often move out of their homes and communities and sometimes to another part of the country that removes them from family, friends, and their community life. While it is possible to stay connected, it is not always easy, especially when experiencing health or cognitive problems.

This can result in feelings of being isolated and removed from the people that comprised their social network. Staying in touch is also made difficult because friendships are usually with those in a similar age group. This means that many of their friends have the same limitations that accompany the aging process, such as declining health and cognitive abilities. In addition, continuing to drive might no longer be an option, further limiting their ability to stay in touch. When that is the case, residents become dependent on friends, family members, or the transportation options available from their CCRC.

Moving into an assisted living community may affect not only the quantity of social relationships but also their quality. One study on assisted living communities and social relationships found that the social relationships healthier residents formed in their ALC with other residents and staff had a more positive effect on life satisfaction than maintaining previous relationships outside the ALC. Residents who are less healthy, mentally and physically, are more likely to experience reduced psychological well-being because they perceive a loss of independence and have less ability to participate socially. This is especially true when residents do not perceive that their community is a good fit for them. They are then less likely to participate in activities offered by the new community or engage with others in social settings, thereby reducing opportunities for experiences that could positively affect their physical and mental health.

New relationships that residents invest in when they move into a CCRC may have a better impact on well-being than previous social relationships. However, life in a CCRC may limit the number of new social relationships; choices for friendship may be limited to the residents residing in the same CCRC. In ALCs, healthier residents have fewer opportunities for new friends. Opportunities are constrained by the higher proportion of mentally and physically infirm residents and therefore fewer activities that can enable social relationships. Even administrative policies that govern something as seemingly innocuous as assigned seating for meals can have consequences in that they can either increase or reduce the options for new relationships. Positive social experiences during meals between residents or between residents and staff can enhance psychological health. Relationships between residents and staff can also offer opportunities for social interaction and friendships, but care-giving staff members are often too busy for developing close relationships with residents. Depending on their age and how healthy they are, they may see their time left as short and thus new friendships that go beyond the surface as being not worth the effort. However, they may not be able to maintain previous close friendships for various reasons such as declining physical and mental health (for both parties) as well as the lack of transportation or distance. This can make residents feel isolated, lonely, and removed from society. Studies that have examined computer and Internet use as a way of moderating the negative effects of relocation on older adults have found a positive relationship between computer and Internet use and quality-of-life outcomes.

2.4   Older adults and technology usage

Some form of technology use is almost a necessity to navigate daily life; those who have limited or no technology experience are at a great disadvantage because it limits their ability to be full participants in an increasingly technological society. Usage of the computer and the Internet has grown substantively among older adults over the past 15 years. As described in Chapter 1, usage among older adults is growing faster than any other age group. It is often assumed that older adults have no interest in learning to use technology. However, this is not necessarily true; they *are* interested in using and have a desire to learn to use technology if they see the relevance of it to their lives and appropriate training is provided.

The number of older adults using computers and the Internet and how often they report using the technology continues to increase. However, older adults aged 76 and older are less likely to use computers and the Internet compared to those under 76. Computer and Internet use declines as age increases, indicative of an age-related digital divide. However, nonuse does not necessarily imply that an older adult has never used a computer, but may simply mean that he or she is not currently using the technology. Nonuse may be related to some type of cognitive or physical condition that makes continuance of usage too difficult or it may be due to individual characteristics whereby the older adult is unwilling to continue usage. It may be that the older adult has no access to a computer or the Internet.

For older adults in CCRCs, the usage and ownership statistics may actually be much lower. The average age of an assisted living resident is 86.9 years, making it much less likely for such a resident to have ever used a computer or the Internet or own any device that has the capacity to access the Internet. CCRC residents face many aging-related physical, emotional, and cognitive changes that can also inhibit computer and Internet usage; the reasons for their transition are often the result of these age-related changes.

Many studies have found the value of both computer and Internet use by older adults as a means of increasing well-being and quality of life (see the list of suggested readings at the end of this chapter). Older computer users utilize the technology most often to make contact and stay in touch with their family and social networks. Unfortunately, for this CCRC population, not only is availability and access to computers and the Internet limited for many, but also many older adults lack any technology experience. The advent of the computer age debuted just as many current older adults were in the process of retiring. Many of them did not use computers in their work or had limited experience with specific, work-related programs. For those in some form of residential care who do not use computers or the Internet, this lack of technology use can increase the perception that they are not a part of the modern, technology-dependent world and have, in effect, been left behind by the rest of society. Potentially, this can impact the quality of life for these older adults.

The benefits of technology for residents in long-term care as a means of staying connected to the world were being examined as early as 1973. Whereas older adults in CCRCs may experience a sense of both social and physical distance, a lack of technology use may add a third layer of separation from modern society. In their study of older adults and computer/Internet use, Richardson, Zorn, and Weaver (2002, p. 17) found that residents in CCRCs who had become computer and Internet users described their feelings as "keeping pace with the modern world," and not "being left behind" by modern society.

The transition into some form of continuing care potentially increases feelings of being too old to learn. This can impact older adults' sense of confidence in their ability to learn something new, such as how to use technology. They may not believe that the benefits they will receive are worth the effort needed to learn the technology. They must be convinced that the value of what they will learn is worth the effort expended in the learning process, whether the barriers to learning are irrational or real.

Lack of access to a computer is a primary reason that older adults do not use the Internet. Not owning a computer or having Internet access is a primary reason that older adults report such a high level of nonuse. Only 48% of older adults over the age of 65 report that they own a desktop computer and about a third report ownership of a laptop. Although Internet access is available through other types of mobile devices, again, the number of older adults reporting ownership of a mobile phone or a tablet computer is low. Tablet computer ownership and use is increasing faster than traditional desktop and laptop computers among older adults.

2.4.1   Barriers to usage among older adults in a CCRC

When older adults move into the CCRC, perceptions of themselves as old, especially in terms of the learning process, may become enhanced. Such perceptions may be especially salient when older adults have the opportunity to learn how to use technology. Their negative perceptions can be overcome, but older adults must be convinced that what they will receive from using the technology is worth the effort of overcoming perceived barriers to use, such as being too old to learn. Technology use in the context of a CCRC allows residents to stay in touch with family and friends and achieve feelings of connection beyond their physical community, thus improving their quality of life. Using a computer and the Internet is an effective tool in overcoming both social barriers (removal from social networks) and spatial barriers (physical distance from previous homes and communities) that are often experienced by older adults who move into a CCRC. Various aspects of well-being have been shown to improve when older adults learn to use computers and the Internet; studies have shown the efficacy of usage in aspects of well-being, such as maintaining important social ties, increasing perceptions of productivity and better cognitive functioning, and higher self-esteem. Even for older adults in the higher age brackets, such as those over 80 years old, using ICTs can help them with social stimulation and connection.

There is a diversity of mental health benefits of ICT use for older adults, which include reduced loneliness, lessened feelings of depression, lowered perceived stress, increased perceptions of personal growth and achievement of individual goals, and renewed feelings of independence, especially for residents who had to transition into a CCRC because of some circumstance beyond their control. Using the computer and Internet is beneficial to older adults in general, but it may be especially beneficial to older adults with some form of disability. It enables them to feel less isolated, providing a virtual means of connection to friends and family, and has the potential to provide a tool for virtual performance of daily tasks, such as shopping or banking.

Technology use can also be useful for enabling older adults removed from former life roles to present and maintain identity when they move away from home into a CCRC.

Technology potentially can play a role in redefining and reshaping attitudes about the meaning of place, so that removal from place is not tantamount to losing identity. Although a CCRC can present attributes of home that allows residents to form an attachment to a new "home," using the Internet offers a means of transcending place and connecting with modern society.

2.4.2   *Technology use and connection to modern society*

Technology use has the potential to integrate older adults into society not only as participants in the culture of technology, but also more fully as participants in broader society. It provides them with opportunities that can be social as well as economic. As discussed previously, it is well documented that the move into a CCRC, especially an assisted living or a skilled nursing facility, often produces an increase in feelings of social and spatial isolation. Therefore, exclusion from technology use becomes yet another level of feeling detached from others and broader society. In many ways, it represents an exclusion from information, especially in the information-based society of today. Residents are excluded from the abundance of digital information that is available to others if they lack access or training or have a condition that inhibits technology use. They find themselves in a "technological catch 22." Because of their age and health status, they stand to benefit greatly from technology use. Yet, it may be precisely because of their age and health status that they do not use technology.

The exclusion from information may inhibit participating in other aspects of society, including political, economic, and cultural aspects, because of the global use of the Internet as the premier information resource. Over time, this will become even more problematic as technology use is necessitated by practically every part of life. Many of the "younger old" adults have had limited exposure to technology and thus may be impacted as they transition into some level of continuing care over the next decade. Beyond the social implications, lack of full access to health information could be a product of nonuse or limited use or access.

One study examined how older women perceive the association between modern society and modern technology (Rosenthal, 2008). The older women in the study who used a computer and the Internet described their usage as an avenue to stay connected to the modern world. Other researchers have found that while it is generally believed that technology use by older adults in various forms of continuing care is both an essential and necessary component of well-being for older adults, it is, sadly, not often a part of their lives.

Older adults can feel a sense of detachment from the modern world and perceive that they are not able to become a part of that world. To them it is unfamiliar and intimidating; they do not see themselves as having the capacity to join the rest of society. They may believe they are too old to learn or may not see the usefulness of technology for where they are in life. Because of the difficulties in learning associated with many aspects of the aging process, they may not believe the benefits outweigh the effort expended in the learning process.

The discomfort residents of CCRCs might feel in learning about or using the Internet may make it more difficult for them to see the necessity and prospective uses of computers and the Internet. The belief they no longer possess the mental acuity required for learning, and especially something that they have no previous context for, can increase their sense of detachment from the process of learning. Feelings of alienation can occur when older adults, who have chosen to avoid usage, are around younger users for whom usage is a necessary and constant part of their life.

Programs that are designed with the challenges and limitations faced by older adults in mind can be effective in helping them to overcome their perceptions of being too old to learn something new. They can, and do, learn to become successful and proficient computer and Internet users. Older adults in continuing care can feel part of the modern world and stay up-to-date with world happenings and changes in addition to staying connected to family and friends. Use of the Internet can potentially help older adults in long-term care feel up-to-date with what is going on in the world outside their CCRC and expose them to new ideas and opportunities, as well as allowing them a means of keeping in touch with others. Technology offers CCRC residents the opportunity to become active participants rather than detached observers.

Recommended readings

More about CCRCs

Caffrey, C., Sengupta, M., Park-Lee, E., Moss, A., Rosenoff, E., and Harris-Kojetin, L. 2012. *Residents living in residential care facilities: United States, 2010* (NCHS Data Brief 91). Hyattsville, Maryland: National Center for Health Statistics.

Cutchin, M. P., Owen, S. V., and Chang, P.-F. J. 2003. Becoming "at home" in assisted living residences: Exploring place integration processes. *Journals of Gerontology: Social Sciences, 58B*(4), S234–S243.

Dupuis-Blanchard, S., Neufeld, A., and Strang, V. R. 2009. The significance of social engagement in relocated older adults. *Qualitative Health Research, 19*(9), 1186–1195.

Eckert, J. K., Carder, P. C., Morgan, L. A., Frankowski, A. C., and Roth, E. G. 2009. *Inside assisted living: The search for home.* Baltimore, Maryland: Johns Hopkins University Press.

Heisler, E., Evans, G. W., and Moen, P. 2003. Health and social outcomes of moving to a continuing care retirement community. *Journal of Housing for the Elderly, 18*(1), 5–23.

Marsden, J. 2005. *Humanistic designs of assisted living.* Baltimore, Maryland: Johns Hopkins University Press.

Sloane, P. D., Zimmerman, S., and Walsh, J. F. 2001. The physical environment. In S. Zimmerman, P. D. Sloane, and J. K. Eckert (Eds.), *Assisted living: Needs, practices and policies in residential care for the elderly* (pp. 173–197). Baltimore, Maryland: Johns Hopkins University Press.

Wilson, K. B. 2007. Historical evolution of assisted living in the United States, 1979 to the present. *The Gerontologist, 47*(Suppl 1), 8–22.

Yamasaki, J. and Sharf, B. F. 2011. Opting out and fitting in: How residents make sense of assisted living and cope with community life. *Journal of Aging Studies, 23*, 13–21.

Zarem, J. E. 2010. *Today's continuing care retirement community (CCRC).* LeadingAge and American Seniors Housing Association. Retrieved from https://www.leadingage.org/uploadedFiles/Content/Consumers/Paying_for_Aging_Services/CCRCcharacteristics_7_2011.pdf

Technology use among older adults

Namazi, K. H., and McClintic, M. 2003. Computer use among elderly persons in long-term care facilities. *Educational Gerontology, 29*(6), 535–550.

Wagner, N., Hassanein, K., and Head, M. 2010. Computer use by older adults: A multi-disciplinary review. *Computers in Human Behavior, 26*, 870–882.

Winstead, V., Anderson, W. A., Yost, E. A., Cotten, S. R., Warr, A., and Berkowsky, R. W. 2013. You can teach an old dog new tricks: A qualitative analysis of how residents of senior living communities may use the web to overcome spatial and social barriers. *Journal of Applied Gerontology, 32*(5), 540–560.

chapter three

A prototype study

3.1 The idea for the study

When the lead author (Shelia Cotten) was a faculty member at the University of Maryland, Baltimore County (UMBC), she became interested in how different generational groups used computers and the Internet. One spring day in 2005, she was contacted by an older man who was interested in the potential of laptop computers to help older adults stay connected with others. He invited her to visit a Jewish retirement community in Maryland where he had been doing some volunteer work with older adults. She visited the community, met the man who had contacted her, and talked with a couple of people he had worked with. The individuals residing at this retirement community reported learning how to use the computer with assistance from others. They reported playing games, searching for information, and using email to write to their family members. Dr. Cotten wondered if teaching older adults in different types of retirement communities to use computers on a larger scale would be possible and feasible. She began to investigate what was known about older adults and technology use in preparation for planning the study detailed in this chapter. After doing much research, meeting with various administrators in different types of communities, and learning a great deal about older adults and the health issues many of them experienced, she pursued funding from the National Institute on Aging to conduct a randomized controlled trial to determine whether computer training for older adults in assisted living communities could positively enhance their quality of life. Funding was received in 2009, and the 5-year project began.

Although our experience and insight comes from within the context of a 5-year research study, the lessons learned are applicable for designers who want to develop and introduce new products, policymakers who recognize the value of large-scale technology interventions, facility managers who want their residents to benefit from technology use, and anyone attempting to implement technology instruction/intervention programs within CCRCs. In some ways, if it is possible to do this type of program within the constraints of a funded research study, with all the attendant rules and requirements, it is certainly possible, and perhaps easier, to do so without such constraints. As this chapter details, we were able to conduct multiple 8-week technology training programs for older adults in CCRCs while coming from outside the organization, having few examples to follow, being constrained (once they were finalized) to our existing materials and assessments, and using what today seems like outdated, oversized, and not very user-friendly technology. The information gleaned through preparing and implementing this trial was substantial. In this and other chapters of this book, we present key considerations for others who wish to implement interventions and trainings in similar contexts.

3.2   Gaining entrance

One of the first and most crucial steps in conducting an intervention or training program is gaining entrance to the communities in which the project will take place. Administrators and activity directors must see the value in your training program for their residents before they will grant you access to their communities. And, if you are testing the efficacy of a particular device, training program, or other technological tool, it will often be necessary to test out these materials in a range of different communities to effectively discern whether and when they produce the outcomes being examined. To gain access to communities, preparation is key.

During the preparation phase, we reached out to all the assisted living communities within 2 hours of Birmingham, Alabama (Dr. Cotten moved to the University of Alabama, Birmingham [UAB] from UMBC in August 2005). At times, it was hard to get our foot in the door at some communities. It is critical to be able to connect with people in charge in the communities to gain their buy-in for your activities. They have to see the value that your project will bring to their residents and the impact that it will have on their communities. They can also aid in connecting you to the best people in the specific communities to help ensure the success of your program. Oftentimes, the CEOs, administrators, owners, and so forth are very busy and may not be easily available to meet with you.

In times like these, it is important to have someone who can help connect you with top administrators in the communities you are hoping to partner with. We were fortunate to have someone who was well connected with many of the communities in the greater Birmingham, Alabama, area. The initial contact for some of the communities was facilitated by Dr. Richard Allman, at that time the director of the UAB Center for Aging. Many of the communities had a good relationship with the Center for Aging; thus, an introduction from Dr. Allman helped to open the doors for our working with them.

We identified all communities that had 40 or more residents, a criterion chosen because we needed to have a sufficient number of potential participants at each site for the intervention. The majority of these communities expressed interest in the study, and many wrote letters of support when the initial grant proposal was submitted to the National Institutes of Health (National Institute on Aging [NIA]) for funding.

After the study was funded, we recontacted the communities to determine whether they were still interested in participating in the randomized controlled trial. We visited the communities to meet with directors, CEOs, activity directors, and other key personnel who helped make decisions about allowing outside entities to conduct community events. We randomized the communities that were interested in participating into three groups: (1) the ICT training group of communities; (2) the attention control group of communities, which comprised communities that received the same level of interaction as the ICT group through activities other than ICT training; and (3) a true control group of communities to which only a survey (which was identical to a survey participants in the other two groups received) was administered.

We conducted the project activities in waves to control, in part, for timing effects. This is most important when conducting research or comparison studies; it is of less concern for deployment of a technology or implementation of an intervention. For instance, we conducted the specific activities within all three groups during the same 8 weeks (e.g., an ICT training, an attention control activity, and true control community receiving only the survey), as close together in time as was feasible given project personnel and community constraints. Once the activities and assessments were completed for the three groups of communities, we began working with a second wave of communities, one from each group. This method of working continued until we completed the study. By conducting all three groups at the same time, we could attempt to control for any events occurring at a local, regional, or national level that might affect the groups.

3.3   Selecting the right context

There are multiple levels of care within CCRCs. It is important to consider which types of participants and which aspects of CCRCs are most important for your project as these choices will affect a multitude of decisions on how to best implement your project.

Although initially we had planned to conduct the training program in assisted living communities, during the pilot of our training program, we realized that individuals in assisted living were frailer than we expected. Some of the potential participants had significant health issues that prevented them from being able to participate in training sessions that each lasted 1.5 hours. For instance, some could not sit this long. Others had significant decline in either physical or cognitive ability that limited their potential participation. The frailty of the potential population is important to consider as it will affect how many have an interest in your project as well as the number who may be physically or cognitively intact enough to effectively complete the program. These factors will also affect specific types of modifications that you may need to make to the setup of your training location, the number of people needed to help facilitate the program, and expected completion rates of participants (some of these issues are discussed later in this chapter). Our experience indicates that cognitive issues are more of a barrier to effective participation than are physical limitations, mainly due to limitations in recall of information being taught to participants that they need to use in future sessions.

Dr. Cotten reached out to assisted living experts around the country and discussed this situation with them. They helped to confirm that the population in assisted living was frailer at that time than had been the case historically. With the societal push to "age in place," many older adults were waiting longer to move into CCRCs. When they did finally move into assisted living communities, in particular, they were frailer than they had been even a decade earlier. And, rather than moving from assisted living communities into other settings offering more skilled nursing care, a larger number of older adults were dying while still residing in assisted living communities.

With this knowledge, Dr. Cotten gained permission from NIA to expand the population of the study to include residents of both assisted and independent living communities. Many of the assisted living communities originally contacted about the project were part of CCRCs, so there was not a need to begin anew with the majority of the communities that would be involved in the study.

3.4   Preparation

Preparing for any sort of classroom teaching experience can be daunting. It can be especially so when the students are not only unfamiliar with the subject matter but also lack the tools or skills necessary to succeed. In the case of technology-training classes for older adults in CCRCs, the ultimate goal was to allow them to be able to use ICTs in a meaningful way. Acquisition of the requisite technological skills was an important step along the way, but definitely not an end unto itself. Because of this, much thought was given to categorizing ICT knowledge into what participants needed to learn to accomplish the goals of the study; what would be nice for them to know, but not necessary for them to succeed; and what would be left out altogether to avoid confusion and overly burdensome detail.

Our reviews of existing training and self-education materials led us to believe that most of what we saw was overly detailed or overly simplistic. For example, to communicate with friends and family using social media, it was not necessary to understand the technical details of how computers communicate across the Internet or how the innards of a computer worked. On the other hand, we also did not want to go too far in the opposite direction by avoiding correct terminology in favor of simplistic explanations. For example, describing the main box of a desktop computer as "the CPU" or the "the hard drive" without acknowledging that, in addition to the CPU and hard drive, it also contained the power supply, the video card or circuitry, and the computer memory would have been too devoid of details. We hoped that this would avoid later confusion with someone saying something like "my hard drive crashed" when all they really knew or meant was that the computer had stopped working. There is a fine line between too much and too little information. We had to be careful not to insult participants by providing too little information and not overwhelm them by providing too much information.

With that in mind, we created our own training manual that focused on the basics of what we felt would be needed to successfully navigate email, the World Wide Web, social media, and entertainment sites. The manual focused on user-level basics, provided plenty of repetition, had illustrative screenshot pictures, and offered clear, concise instructions and annotated illustrations. Each manual was personalized for each participant, produced in full color, and bound in a three-ring, eight-tab binder (one tab for each weekly lesson) to allow for easily adding note pages to the manual itself, a feature many participants took advantage of. See Table 3.1 for a list of the contents of the training manual. A more detailed listing of the contents of the training manual is included in the Appendix.

Well before the beginning of the training session, a site visit was necessary to assure that everything that would be needed was in place. During a site visit, we assessed space, scheduling, and logistics (each of which is addressed in more detail later), as well as Internet connectivity

Table 3.1 Training manual table of contents

Introduction	
Week 1	The basics of the computer as a tool
Week 2	You won't need a letter opener for email
Week 3	Introducing the Internet
Week 4	Some more email goodness
Week 5	Advanced Internet—getting social on the Web
Week 6	Making sense of the Internet
Week 7	The entertaining Internet
Week 8	Wrapping up
	Glossary
	Step-by-step guides

and electrical connections. During these site visits, it was critical to bring the actual equipment that would be used and make sure that the Internet connections that would be available were reliable and capable of handling the traffic that would be generated by the class. In several instances, this was not the case and connections needed either to be added or upgraded. Determining this far ahead of time reduced or eliminated the need to cancel or reschedule.

Another concern was electrical outlets. Some spaces we identified did not have enough electrical outlets to support the class. Although we were using laptop computers, they often still required being plugged in to maintain power for the duration of the class. The number of outlets needed was determined not only by the number of computers that would be used in class but also the layout of the room. As we discuss in further detail later, making up for poorly placed outlets by using extension cords is not always a wise option.

Aside from ensuring that the space was appropriate for a class, we also made sure our equipment was ready for each class. This involved wiping and reimaging (erasing and reinstalling a standard software setup) on each laptop prior to the beginning of each new series of training sessions. Over the course of training sessions, settings could be changed, items could be downloaded to the laptop, and, in some cases, viruses or malware could find their way onto the computers. The reimaging process ensured that we started each round of training sessions from a standardized starting point in terms of software, options, and settings. Because of our desire for a customized experience, we also created unique logins for each participant and labeled each computer with a participant's name. In addition to creating a customized experience, this also allowed us to make sure that each participant got the same computer each class, thus assuring that any customizations remained in place. For ease of administration, however, the image used to reimage each computer had all the customized login credentials for the entire class—only one computer had Mr Smith's name on it, but, in actuality, Mr Smith could have logged into any computer in the class using his same login and password. This also allowed us to easily replace any computer that was malfunctioning.

3.4.1   Assistive devices

Key considerations when working with older adults are issues involving hearing, vision, and motor control. Hearing and vision issues are perhaps obvious. Rigging the instructor with a microphone and providing large screens or vision assistive software were adequate to address most vision and hearing problems.

Motor control issues may be less obvious, but more difficult to overcome. Most of us may take moving the mouse and double-clicking for granted, but such movements require a level of control that many older adults may no longer possess. Holding a mouse completely still while simultaneously using a finger to press a button on the mouse is an underappreciated feat of fine motor control. If you have ever slipped up during this process, you can understand how easy it can be to make an errant click and end up attempting to rename a file or dumping a desktop icon into another folder or the trash. We found that a large trackball (Figure 3.1) was often the best option in these cases. It allowed participants to position the pointer using the ball, leave the ball in place, and then click as a separate operation. We also, found, however, that many participants were hesitant to use these devices, telling us that they "didn't need anything like that." Often, this seemed to be indicative of some embarrassment over needing special consideration or denial that motor control might be an issue. In these cases, we would often install a large trackball any way and ask them just to try it for a couple of minutes. Most participants in these situations liked the trackball and continued to use it.

Another assistive device was a large-key keyboard in either a QWERTY or alphabetical configuration. Such keyboards offered three advantages. First, their one-inch-square keys with large lettering were very easy to see and read, helping those with vision problems. Second, the large keys made it easier for those with motor control issues to press the key they intended to press. Third, the alphabetical keyboard was much easier to use for "hunt and peck" typists who were unfamiliar with the QWERTY layout.

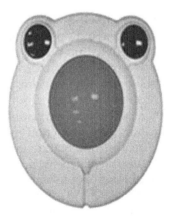

Figure 3.1 Large trackball.

3.4.2   Recruiting

Recruiting was done through formal recruiting sessions. With the help of CCRC administrators and activities directors, we would schedule and publicize recruiting events where our staff would present an overview of the study, demonstrate some of the equipment, and take questions. The style of these events varied from location to location. At some locations, they were more formal, where we would stand at the front of a room with a slide show projected onto a screen behind us. We would talk about the study, handing off the presentation to different team members to cover different aspects of the training. At others, we presented at community meetings, spoke informally with smaller groups, or even had more elaborate events to coincide with other community events. For example, in one community, we provided refreshments for and spoke at a community event that involved music and dancing, staying to mingle with the residents and answer questions. None of these seemed to be particularly more successful than the others; however, there were three things that we noted that were especially useful in recruiting.

We felt more at home and more accepted as part of the community when we mixed with other events and took time to mingle with the residents and answer questions. On the other hand, we took it as a lesson learned that recruitment during community meetings was not the best idea. At some of these meetings, residents or their family members may be airing grievances or other presenters may be talking at some length about matters that no one is interested in hearing about or discussing. If your recruitment precedes these, they will kill a lot of the momentum or interest you may have generated. If your recruitment follows these, you may find yourself in an awkward situation of trying to sound upbeat while talking about an exciting new opportunity just after hearing how residents are fed up with the dining options in their community.

Finally, although stand-alone events were much better than those associated with serious business, associating our recruitment with some sort of celebration or other upbeat activity, had the double advantage of catching residents when they were in a good mood and when more of them were likely to have turned out. Stand-alone events attracted only those who were intrinsically interested, whereas hybrid recruitment—CCRC activity events brought out people who might otherwise not have bothered to attend.

Whatever the style of the event, we felt that it was essential to bring equipment and materials with us to demonstrate. Many of our participants who were at first skeptical were sold on participating (based on their comments) after glancing through the training manual, playing with a large-key keyboard or large trackball, or seeing the size of the computer screens and some of the things we would be covering in the class. Part of this is what made the hybrid recruiting events a better option—we could reach those who otherwise would have written off a computer class as something they could not participate in or would not find interesting.

3.5 Staging the intervention: where, when, and how to set up the training sessions

3.5.1 Where: find lots of room

We found the three most important considerations when deciding where to stage the training sessions to be having (1) ample room, (2) little noise and few distractions, and (3) easy access for both the trainers and participants.

First, the location must provide ample room for the class to be conducted. Of course, this includes the room needed for each participant with his or her equipment and materials (about 3–4 feet of table space), but also room for training assistants to move around freely. Sometimes the location was set up as a fairly traditional classroom, with long tables set 4–6 feet apart to allow us to move up and down the rows. In other locations, long tables were not available, and square or round tables had to be used. In these cases, usually no more than two people could be placed at a table (although sometimes three could be squeezed in). This arrangement requires more space per participant, however. Because participants are not side by side, space is required for training assistants to move around both behind tables and between tables. Figure 3.2 shows one of our training rooms.

The room should be set up in such a way as to allow larger open spaces near the entrance to the room for participants who may require the use of wheelchairs or scooters. In a similar vein, preference for the locations closest to the main instructor should be given to participants who may have hearing or vision problems. Although the issues with hearing may be overcome by use of a microphone, the only real solution for participants who have difficulty seeing the instructor's screen is to have them sit near the front. For this reason, consideration must also be given to the placement of a screen, projector, or large screen TV. In cramped spaces, a projected image may not be large enough or high enough up to be seen by those near the back of the class.

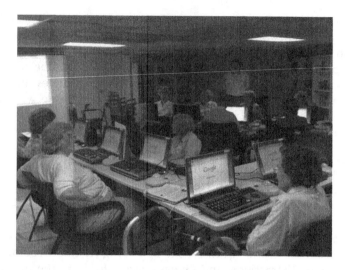

Figure 3.2 Photo of a training room layout.

Wiring is an important consideration. Although we were using laptops with extra capacity batteries, as they aged, they were unable to last through a session, requiring us to always plug in the computers. Therefore, we needed room to run extension cords, power strips, and power supplies in a way that was unobtrusive and out of the way so that participants would not become tangled in them or trip. In some locations, this meant setting up the room and then disconnecting the power (i.e., unplugging and stowing extension cords or power strips) until all participants were seated, so that we could then rerun the power cords.

In sum, the more room, the better. Of course, these are ideal circumstances. Although we never considered any space too large, we often found spaces to be too small or otherwise poorly configured for class. Still, we found ways to make do. For example, some room configurations we experienced required us to station our assistants in parts of a room where they would be "trapped" until class was over because tables or participant seating blocked the way. Other locations required participant seating arranged according to the need for assistive devices; for example, those needing an external mouse or trackball might be required to sit in one area of the room where there was more space to spread out, while those who were comfortable with the built-in trackpad would sit in other areas where the seating could be more closely spaced. Likewise, the trainer sometimes was located more in the middle of the participants rather than clearly out in front. Taken together, these experiences highlight the necessity of being flexible in setting up equipment and arranging people and seating. No two rooms and no two cohorts of participants will be the same. Acknowledging this and adapting to the people and circumstances are key to a successful outcome.

In addition to having ample space for participants, equipment, and trainers, noise and distractions are also important considerations. In our experience, large open areas that would provide the space necessary to conduct the classes were oftentimes also near high-traffic areas or were high-traffic areas themselves. Several times we set up the classes in areas that brought us spectators and passers-by. This was usually not much of a problem, but sometimes could be. More often than not, residents who were not participating would either notice the class in session and be unobtrusive, perhaps pulling an assistant aside to ask what was going on; however, on occasion, a resident would interrupt the class to find out what was happening or to ask to join, even late into the sessions.

In some locations, dining areas are often attractive options for holding a larger class. They offer ample space for participants (plenty of space for each participant, along with room for assistants to move around) and ease of setup (tables and chairs were already in place). Sometimes dining areas may be the only areas large enough to accommodate technology-training classes. Our training configuration (an 18.5-inch laptop, external keyboard, and mouse or trackball, along with a place for the training manual and notepad) took quite a bit of space to fit in comfortably. Although dining rooms often had the space we needed, they offered their own difficulties.

In addition to working around the actual meal service, we also had to work around dining room preparation and cleaning, as well as residents who were eager for mealtime and would sometimes come in, take their usual mealtime places, and begin conversations, interrupting the class. Dining staff might also interrupt to set tables or otherwise prepare the meal service. So while dining areas may seem like the perfect alternative, they were often severely constrained in terms of the times available for training, a topic we discuss in the next section.

Another regular source of interruption came in spaces that were booked for other events either before or after the training classes. Events beforehand often meant a rush to get set up for class. Events after the class often meant feeling rushed to wrap up and break down or, in some cases, enduring glaring looks and comments from people waiting to get into the room. The ideal, of course, would be a large, quiet, out of the way room that was not booked for any activities prior or subsequent to the training session. We found this to be a very rare option unless the class was very small.

The final consideration for staging the intervention was ease of access for participants and trainers. Perhaps these notes will seem obvious, but locations that are easier to access and set up are preferred over those that are more difficult to access and set up.

In most cases, we asked for space to store our equipment onsite to avoid unnecessary and logistically cumbersome loading, moving, and unloading of equipment, which was stored in locked cases. Often, this storage was near the training location, which made it easy to retrieve the cases and set up the classroom in fairly short order. Other times, however, this was not the case. The worst example had us storing equipment in a basement location that required the use of two separate elevators and extended walks down three long hallways to get the equipment from storage to the classroom. In addition to the long haul and elevators, we often waited to allow residents to use the elevators so as not to be obtrusive. This required arriving at this location at least 45 minutes ahead of the scheduled class time to ensure plenty of time to move equipment and set up the classroom. In total, this was little more than an inconvenience for us, but, if the option is available, closer storage is better. Only once did we actually cancel a class due solely to storage issues. The elevator would not work and the only way around it would have been to take everything out of the rolling cases (which were too heavy to carry when loaded) and carry it by hand up some stairs and down a long hallway, something we did not have time (or strength) to do because we arrived too late, assuming the elevator would work.

In our examples, access refers not only to access to the room itself but also to other things that will be needed, such as tables, chairs, and audiovisual (AV) equipment. In the best instances, there was storage for equipment, tables, chairs, and AV equipment just off the room being used for the training. This made setup quick and easy and allowed for some flexibility should someone insist on joining the class late. What we quickly learned was less desirable were locations where tables and chairs had to be rounded up on a case-by-case basis by someone from the staff or where tables, chairs, equipment, or the room itself were only accessible with the correct keys. On several occasions, although prior arrangements had been made, we found ourselves temporarily unable to access needed space or equipment because the person who had the key was unable to be found.

3.5.2   When: scheduling and fitting into CCRC schedules

For many of the communities in which we worked, regular schedules were as important as any other aspect of the community, with the exception of assistive care. Mealtimes are the backbone of the schedule and were inviolable. Early on, we recognized the importance of mealtimes and the activities associated with them. In addition to ensuring that residents were done with class in time to adhere to the regular meal schedule, many residents wanted to be sure that they would have time to prepare for meals by returning to their rooms to freshen up, to retrieve medications that might need to be taken with a meal, or to retrieve other items they might want to take with them, like books, magazines, or items they wanted to share with other residents. At some locations, mealtime unofficially required a level of attire that participants may not have wanted to wear to a computer training class; thus, allowing time for residents to prepare for mealtime after the training class or to prepare for class after the meal was important.

In at least one location, we often assisted in dining room setup for the lunch service so that it would be ready in time for residents to begin arriving. Even so, we often endured glares from some waiting residents, who preferred to arrive early and read or converse before the lunch was served. Similarly, trying to work the classes in after a meal service can result in the awkward situation of asking residents who may be taking their time to leave or relocate so that the room can be prepared for class. For these reasons, we preferred to avoid dining areas unless we could fit the class in well away from dining times, something more easily accomplished in the early afternoon.

As we discuss further in a later chapter, another thing we learned early on was the importance of established activities at CCRCs. Our shorthand for this was "you don't mess with bingo." Due to its popularity at many locations, we often had to schedule around bingo. Not every resident liked bingo, of course, and many of our study participants would gladly forgo bingo to participate in the training sessions. For those who really liked bingo, however, rescheduling it to accommodate a computer training class was unacceptable. Bingo was the shorthand, but this could be true of other activities as well—bible study, craft groups, beauty shop hours, regularly scheduled shopping trips, and so on. It highlighted for us the need to consider not only the schedules of the people who were participating in the training class but also of everyone who lived in the CCRC. Our participants might be fine with the weekly big box shopping trip being moved to Wednesday to accommodate our Tuesday and Thursday computer class, but many others might not. With this in mind, we tried to go out of our way to fit into whatever time slots would be least disruptive to the CCRC residents, staying late, rescheduling our own classes when possible (in the case of graduate student assistants), or working over our own lunch time.

Ideally, we preferred scheduling classes such that we could have a class early in the week, an office hours session in the middle of the week, and a second class later in the week. Because each week was a unit in itself, this configuration allowed for introduction of new material in the first class, practice and questions during office hours, and reinforcement and presentation of advanced material in the following class. In practice, this configuration was sometimes not possible, with office hours coming between weekly units, rather than between class sessions.

3.5.3   How: reducing distractions and frustrations— making it a good experience

One of our goals was to minimize any fuss or frustration that the participants might experience. We understood that some of the participants were very hesitant and unsure they should even be participating. Frustrations like a chaotic room, malfunctioning equipment, or lack of an assistive device could mean they would withdraw. On the first day of training, it is wise to begin setting up very early, at least 1.5 hours ahead of time, for even small classes. This allows plenty of time to track down tables and chairs if needed, arrange the room as needed, put out all equipment, connect everything, and test everything out before participants arrive. Many participants will arrive early and will be eager to be seated at a computer. If you want to avoid asking people to move or wait while you finish the setup, it is best to get started very early. Some participants may also want to help with the setup. While we always sincerely appreciated the offer, the setup went more quickly when we politely declined the help.

Setting up the training classroom is quite different from simply taking out a laptop and putting it on a table. After a few sessions, we began to learn what did and did not work in terms of setup and had our own particular techniques to make sure cables were out of the way and each participant had enough space. We would also produce seating charts after participants settled into their "regular" seats. We noted on these charts the preferences of each participant in terms of assistive devices, left/right handedness, and so on. This allowed us to have everything in place before participants arrived, rather than having to ask at each session.

After the first couple of sessions, classes usually settle into a routine, and the equipment setup can begin as late as half an hour prior to the session if the room has been set up ahead of time. Our preferred sequence was to arrange the room first, set up the instructor's computer, projector, and screen, put out the laptops (including power supplies), and then add any extra devices needed by participants. Still, adaptability and flexibility are key. We always had on hand (unless the class was very large) more of everything than what we expected to use (e.g., more assistive devices [see Table 3.2], extra copies of the manual, backup Wi-Fi router, backup projector, and extra laptops). Thus, if a laptop began having problems, we had extra laptops that we could quickly boot up, bring to the current point in the lesson (e.g., get to a search results page), and then simply swap out for the malfunctioning laptop. If a participant who never used a

Table 3.2 Assistive devices

Device	Advantage
Large trackball	A large trackball increases the ease of interacting with a mouse. The large ball allows a participant to more easily move the pointer as desired and it allows for easier fine control of the pointer position. The participant can then click without affecting the position of the pointer.
Large-key keyboard	A keyboard with one-inch-square keys that give a definitive "click" when pressed is easier to use by those who may have trouble seeing the keyboard, and it provides greater confidence in use for those unfamiliar with a keyboard. An alphabetically arranged version is a good option for those unfamiliar with the QWERTY layout.
Large monitors	A larger monitor allows for larger icons and text, improving readability for those with impaired eyesight.
Low vision assistive software	Such software, sometimes combined with a larger screen, greatly aids those with vision difficulties.

large trackball before was having issues with using a mouse, we had extra trackballs on hand so that we could plug one in and let him or her try it.

We also produced backup plans for (what came to seem to be inevitable) issues beyond our control. For example, one location routinely had Internet connection trouble, a real problem if you are trying to teach participants to use email. On those days, we would use prepared screenshots to illustrate what the actual email composition screen would look like and had participants type their messages using Notepad. On other days, we might work in more mouse or keyboard practice. On still other occasions, we might create our own Internet connections by using our smartphones as Wi-Fi hotspots.

Even with weeks of preparation, testing of Wi-Fi and electrical connections, a well-planned room setup, and even after gaining experience conducting the intervention in several locations, the first couple of training sessions will always bring surprises— new participants, changes in Internet access, last minute relocations, and getting participants settled in generally. All this is to say that being ready for things not to go quite as planned should be part of the preparation.

3.6   Implementation

Because our manual had been carefully designed, we followed the manual as closely as possible. The first session usually began with making sure that everyone was comfortable, could see and hear well, and was ready to begin.

All sessions included a lead trainer and a number of assistants who were stationed throughout the room. The lead trainer was responsible for leading the class, moving through the session materials, demonstrating procedures on the screen, answering class questions, and, during time meant for participants to work individually or in small groups, moving around the room with the assistants to help participants and answer questions. The assistants were stationed throughout the room, primarily taking responsibility for a particular area and number of participants, but more generally assisting anyone who needed help. One of the assistants was always the designated tech support person who was called over to help if there was a computer or Internet problem.

The lead instructor must be comfortable with speaking slowly and clearly and be willing to repeat explanations and instructions many times. This may seem obvious, but we found that some staff were uncomfortable with the rate of speech and amount of repetition required to be a good lead instructor. Our best lead instructor perfected an air of calm assurance that translated well for participants, the instructor's demeanor and tone helping them feel that it was acceptable to make mistakes and learn from them. We found that rushed, impatient, or otherwise unsympathetic instructors could quickly turn a class session into a trying experience for many participants. Unlike other settings where perhaps the participants could learn on their own, despite a less than optimal instructor, in the CCRC setting, most participants relied heavily on the instructor to help them understand the material. Feeling okay about not understanding and receiving some patient, sympathetic help was practically as important as the material itself in helping participants to progress.

Because we were working from few existing examples, training for our instructors consisted more of trial and error and mock sessions rather than formal training sessions. As much as is possible, you should ensure that there is standardization across multiple instructors. As our team had worked together quite extensively by the time we began our intervention, lack of standardization was less of an issue than it may be for others.

Although our approach may not seem ideal, we actually see great value in this approach. Though we were constrained by needing to follow the same protocol and procedures each time, those not conducting a study can feel free to try new approaches and presentations in an attempt to better reach each new participant or cohort. This is to say, it is probably wise to worry less about having a formally trained instructor than it is to enlist someone with the requisite technology knowledge and experience, and who also has the demeanor and attitude necessary to interact comfortably and easily with older adults who may be reticent, skeptical, or even hostile toward new technology. Unless you are conducting a research study, worry less about training and consistency and more about human connection and adaptation to the circumstances. However, if the same instructor will not be available for every class meeting, consistency across the instructors becomes more important for the benefit of the participants.

Being an effective assistant also required a calm, assured demeanor and a great deal of patience. Participants who felt rushed or embarrassed by the help they received were at best unlikely to ask for help again, and at worst, were likely to let the instructor and assistants know exactly how they felt. That said, instructors and assistants must strike a balance between being helpful and sympathetic and undermining the training by doing too much for participants. There is a stereotype of the technology support person or instructor who, upon encountering a problem, just moves user or student aside and fixes the problem himself or herself. Although we found ourselves wanting to do that in some situations, we understood that *success depended upon the participants learning to take care of their own problems.* Thus, the first course of action was always to ask the participant what he or she thought needed to be done. The last course of action was to do something for the participant. For example, if a participant was having trouble sending an email, we might notice immediately that the problem was the lack of an address in the "To:" field. Rather than simply saying, "Oh, it looks like you haven't put a recipient address in," we would instead ask such questions as "Okay, let's see, what are the three things we talked about it being good to have in every email?" (i.e., recipient address, subject, and message) or "who are you sending this message to, again?" These kinds of questions usually prompted the participant to notice that they had left off the recipient's address. We would then advise them to add the address and see if that corrected the problem.

Of course, if it became clear that the problem was beyond the scope of the class, then the instructor or assistants would step in and do what needed to be done, telling participants that, for a problem like this, they would need to ask for help from someone who was really good at fixing a computer. Examples of these types of problems included such issues as moderate to major Internet connection problems (e.g., something more serious than, e.g., the Wi-Fi having been switched off), major software problems (e.g., something that could not be cleared by restarting either the program or the computer), or hardware problems more serious than something like a mouse becoming unplugged.

We began and ended each session with an overview of what would be covered, combined with a brief review of the previous session and a review of what had been covered, along with a preview of the next session.

3.7   Retention

With a large-scale project such as the one we conducted, paying attention to participant retention was critical to ensuring the success of our project and that we would have adequate numbers to answer the research questions put forth in the original proposal to NIH. However, even if you do not have to report to a funding agency, retention is important to your efforts because it is the gauge against which you will measure the worth of the program to your participants. Simply put, if your participants are dropping out, it is an indication that they are not finding any benefit from the training. They may be looking for something as simple as an interesting way to spend a few hours each week. They may also be trying to learn the details of how to use the technology so that they can be proficient on their own. The trick for retention is finding the right balance. When the balance is correct, participants will be more likely to keep coming back and to recommend to others that they give it a try. The wrong balance, making things overly technical or difficult, or having a poor instructor, will make it more likely that participants will stop coming and will also discourage others from ever starting. Still, whatever balance you strike (and that will depend on the makeup of each training cohort), there are some strategies to encourage retention in any situation.

To encourage retention, we employed a number of different approaches. Many of these involved being supportive and responsive to the needs of our participants. Within the scope of the project, we tried to engage participants in as many aspects of the training as possible. For example, when we had to search for materials on the Internet, we asked them for topics. When covering entertainment sites such as Hulu and YouTube, we asked participants to name a singer that they enjoyed listening to. Often this would be someone who was popular 30–50 years ago. Participants were amazed at the range of singers and television shows that could be found online, including ones from their generation. Getting participants excited about what they were learning meant they stayed engaged in the training program.

A larger approach is simply getting to know each participant and understanding what he or she wants from the class. Most participants will sit through an occasional session that does not interest them or material that they find confusing or irrelevant if the trainers demonstrate an understanding that this is the case for them and attempt to offer something indicating this. For example, you may approach a participant at the end of a class and let them know that the next session is something that they had said they were not interested in, but that you encourage them to come because you have tried to include a couple of skills or pieces of information that they may find useful. Similarly, you might attempt to tailor some of the sessions in a way that you still cover the material you wished to cover, but in a way that incorporates some specific interests.

Within the larger scope of our project, we were also able to tailor the training in some cases. For example, although we introduced the topic of social networking sites in class, few of our participants were interested in joining these sites. Thus, we had the ones who were interested in joining one or more social networking sites attend an office hours where we would show them how to join. As more participants were interested in learning how to effectively use email, we spent more time than originally planned with this aspect of the training, compared to time spent on social networking sites.

Even though being responsive and attentive to our participants helped to reduce attrition and maintain retention, there were times when nothing we could do could help with these issues. As is typical with older adults in CCRCs, there are usually health issues that led many of them to move into these communities. We found that as our 8-week training sessions progressed, as well as the year-long follow-up after the training, a percentage of our participants experienced significant health issues that resulted in their not being able to continue in the training. It was very sad for us to see some of our participants' health decline, and even sadder when some of them tried to rejoin the class but their health (in particular, their memory) would not let them retain the material they had learned.

In addition to health issues, we had some participants who moved to other CCRCs, and a few who passed away. Others were not able to continue due to lack of participation (we had a specific number of classes that participants could miss and still stay in the class) or interest. Although we had 314 participants who passed our cognitive screener (for the full study), by the end of our involvement with participants 12 months past the end of the 8-week sessions, we had only 208 participants who completed the final assessment.

3.8   Assessment

Our experience, of course, was within the context of conducting a research study. Thus, we had specific outcomes related to quality of life, use of computers and the Internet, and so on that we were interested in assessing throughout the course of our study. Even if the training is not being provided in the context of a research study, assessment of progress and outcomes is still important. Participants like to see that they are making progress. Regular assessment throughout the training can help them track progress and realize how much they have learned. Assessment can also help assure you that you are not wasting the residents' or participants' time with something that you find very interesting but that they do not. Regular and adequate assessment will help you avoid this and offer a program that can actually lead to better quality of life for the residents.

As this was a research study funded by NIA, we had specific outcomes that we were examining and that we could not alter during the course of the study. Our assessments were conducted through surveys and focus groups. We developed a survey that we administered prior to the beginning of any project activities, at the end of the 8-week activities, and at 3, 6, and 12 months after the activities. The survey contained a variety of items regarding health, quality of life, computer and Internet use, and attitudes toward technology. Focus group questions concerned the training activities, future intentions to use technology, and perceptions of impacts of using computers and the Internet on various aspects of their lives. Focus groups were conducted at the end of the ICT and attention control activities at each community. In addition to surveys and focus groups, our research team took extensive field notes regarding the training sessions as well as observation notes recorded by all team members at various points throughout the study.

The variety of the assessments used in this project allowed us to examine the range of outcomes of note in our funded proposal, as well as how processes and outcomes changed over the course of the project. Regardless of the entity conducting the training, we recommend having clearly identified expected outcomes of the training and developing research materials to assess whether the outcomes have been met during and as a function of the training. In our case, we also wanted to know whether the effects of the training would persist over time. Determining the larger goals of the project can help determine specific outcomes of interest as well as the correct time frame in which to examine them.

In the case of the CCRC, conducting technology training sessions free from the constraints of research funding and requirements provides the opportunity to make assessments even more meaningful for the instructors and participants. Consider incorporating feedback after each session or unit. Find out what worked, what did not, and what residents want to see and learn. Work with the participants to set not only personal goals for each of them but also larger goals for the overall program. Then, enlist participants in measuring the progress toward those goals. These types of active, participatory assessments will yield a better program for residents, increase feelings of active involvement, and result in better retention and outcomes.

3.9   Lessons learned

Developing a computer training program such as the one described in this chapter is very complex. There are a variety of "actors" involved that affect how such a training program takes place. After conducting our intervention, we learned several lessons that we believe will help others who may wish to implement similar programs in CCRCs.

- Buy-in from the CCRCs is critical to effectively implementing a program.

- Engaged activity directors help to ensure the success of the program because they may have more frequent interaction with the participants and can encourage their continued participation.
- Technology tailored to the participants is important for helping to ensure their success in the training (e.g., having assistive devices when needed).
- Adequate space and resources are critical to the success of the training.
- Helping residents see how learning to use the technology can positively impact their lives is critical to helping them cross the digital divide and learn to effectively use the technology tools.
- Keeping participants engaged is critical to ensuring that they will continue in the program. Helping them see their progression will also help them stay engaged.
- Repetition is important so that older adults have opportunities to practice the skills they are learning. Scaffolding is also important, as they learn to build upon earlier skills they have acquired in the training in order to progress to more advanced activities.
- Having a training manual that corresponds to what they learn in the training and that simplifies training activities helps to reinforce what they are learning.

Whereas this chapter has focused on our specific training intervention project, the next chapter details complexities and best practices for implementing training programs such as this one in CCRCs. Additional literature is included, as well as a list of summary guidelines for those interested in conducting such training programs in CCRCs.

Recommended readings

Czaja, S. J. and Sharit, J. 2013. *Designing training and instructional programs for older adults.* Boca Raton, Florida: CRC Press.

Fisk, A. D., Rogers, W. A., Charness, N., Czaja, S. J., and Sharit, J. 2009. *Designing for older adults: Principles and creative human factors approaches* (2nd ed.). Boca Raton, Florida: CRC Press.

Rogers, W. A. and Fisk, A. D. 2010. Toward a psychological science of advanced technology design for older adults. *The Journals of Gerontology Series B: Psychological Sciences and Social Sciences, 65B*(6), 645–653. http://doi.org/10.1093/geronb/gbq065

chapter four

Complexities of and best practices for implementing technology training in continuing care retirement communities

With the rapid increase in technological advancement as well as the increase in access to and use of technologies such as Internet-connected computers and smartphones, there has been a growth of literature focusing on the best practices in teaching new users how to adequately use a new technology. But although there are now a number of articles and books devoted to tips and tricks associated with teaching someone how to use a computer or the Internet, there is very little that specifically caters to the needs of residents in CCRCs. People who implement training programs in such settings have a number of variables to take into account that people in other technology training situations need not consider, including (but not limited to) setting up a training area that allows enough space for residents and their canes, walkers, or wheelchairs to navigate through; creating a learning environment where residents with visual impairment can easily see their computers as well as the instructor; accommodating individuals with dexterity issues or tremors so that they may use a keyboard or a mouse; scheduling the training sessions around the other activities being conducted at the CCRC; and creating a support system wherein residents may ask questions about technology within the CCRC when the classes are not in session. Considerations like this can bring new challenges to technology trainers hoping to teach CCRC residents how to use new technologies—not just personal computers, but *all* current and emerging ICTs (e.g., smartphones, tablet computers, personal digital assistants, and even Internet-connected television sets). Some of these considerations were touched upon in Chapter 3; here, we dive deeper into the difficulties technology trainers may face.

This chapter outlines special considerations technology instructors and others must take into account when implementing a technology intervention in a CCRC setting. Topics that are addressed include the complexities and best practices associated with understanding the learning needs of the CCRC resident as a student, organizing the learning environment for optimal instruction and a positive classroom experience, ensuring the proper equipment is on hand, designing and presenting the content included in technology lessons, and engaging and motivating class participants. Although the chapter pulls from our experiences conducting ICT classes in assisted living communities and independent living communities (ALCs and ILCs), the best practices outlined can arguably be implemented in other levels of care at a CCRC and can also be used in a wide array of technology classes, not just basic computer or Internet courses.

4.1   Understanding the learner

Let us propose a hypothetical situation: let's say that you are given the task to design and implement a class whose focus is on the history of the 2008 US presidential election. Specifically, you are to list and give brief biographies of the major players in the election (including the presidential candidates and their running mates), give a summary timeline of events leading up to election day, and explain the theories scholars put forth as to how Barack Obama won the election against John McCain. Given the appropriate reference materials and a bit of time, this appears like a very doable task.

Now let us throw a monkey wrench into things: imagine you were given this task only to later learn that the class you will be presenting in is *full of elementary school students*. It is very likely your hypothetical class was designed for a different audience—high school students, college students, or even adults who have already graduated from high school or college. Elementary school students, however, are much younger, have had less educational training, and also have specific learning needs that are vastly different from other groups. In all likelihood, your hypothetical class will no longer work with this audience, and you will have to design a new class that presents the material in a new way younger people can more easily understand.

This hypothetical situation illustrates the importance of understanding the learning needs of those whom you are trying to teach. While the same topics can be taught across different audiences, *how* these topics are covered will vary vastly and will be dependent on necessity, the preferences of the student, and the context. In this section, we highlight some of the learning needs specific to older learners and the considerations that need to be made when implementing technology training for this group, including accounting for physical and cognitive declines and declines in dexterity and visual and hearing ability. Confidence in learning and motivation to learn, and how to engage older adult learners, could also fall under this purview but are discussed in more detail later in this chapter.

4.1.1 Physical health and mobility of older learners

Physical deterioration can make it difficult for older adults to get to and from class without the assistance of a walker, cane, or wheelchair, assuming the class is within walking distance. The difficulties associated with physical health are exacerbated if the class is offsite (i.e., the student needs to travel via car, van, or public transport to attend the class). For CCRC residents, mobility is an important issue as a majority, especially those in assisted living, require some sort of assistive device to help them get from place to place, such as a walker or wheelchair, and thus it can be an overwhelming task for them just to go from room to room, let alone go somewhere outside the CCRC. And even if the resident can leave, transportation to an offsite location can be tricky; not all are able to drive themselves, and not every CCRC has a transport system in place to take residents to different locations.

Therefore, technology trainers need to account for mobility issues. In our study, this meant bringing the class to the residents through the use of a mobile lab. Rather than holding the class in a community center or at a university, we instead took our mobile computer lab and brought it to the CCRC, setting up the class in a room at the CCRC that was easily accessible to the residents (usually a room that they frequented). This meant more work for us (as we were now the ones who were constantly traveling), but by making it easy for residents to get to and from class, participants will have less stress about their ability to get to class and will find the experience all the more comfortable and enjoyable.

Mobility is not the only physical limitation trainers need account for. Comfort in the classroom is another important consideration. Many older adults tend to have a hard time sitting in one place for an extended period of time; sitting in one place (especially without proper support) can lead to pain in the back and legs. Having proper seating can go a long way in preventing pain associated with being seated for an extended period. In our experience, many older adults in CCRCs opt for chairs with high backs (for support) and extra cushioning. Having armrests on the chair can also be advantageous, as many older adults use these to get up and down from a chair.

Illness can also pose as a significant barrier to learning, as older adults tend to be more susceptible to various ailments that can keep them from coming to class. These can range from relatively minor (such as a case of the common cold that keeps them in their room for a day) to more severe (such as pneumonia that sends the resident to the hospital for an extended period). Illness cannot be planned for, but steps can be taken to make sure the sick resident will be able to catch up once he or she is able to attend class again. As a reminder from the previous chapter, in our study, we had optional office hour sessions during our 8-week interventions wherein residents could come in and get one-on-one time with our instructors. For many residents who missed class due to illness, these office hours actually served as a makeup day where they would come in, learn the material they missed, and practice a bit.

For those who wish to conduct technology classes with residents of CCRCs, the takeaways regarding physical health and mobility are as follows:

- Make travel to the class as easy as possible by *bringing the class to the participants*. Hold the class sessions in the CCRC (rather than offsite at a community center) and choose a location for the class that is easily accessible. Popular locations tend to be dining halls or activity rooms.
- *Choose a room that makes mobility in the class easy*, with enough space for furniture (tables and chairs) but also enough open space so that participants with walkers or wheelchairs may easily maneuver.
- *Cater the seating to the physical and comfort needs of the class* (e.g., provide chairs with more cushioning for those who need them, and high tables for those sitting in motorized wheelchairs).
- Have a plan to *accommodate those who miss class due to illness* (e.g., provide makeup sessions or include optional office hours in your class protocol).

4.1.2   Dexterity and visual and hearing ability

Trainers must accommodate older adults' limitations in dexterity and visual and hearing ability. A wealth of research literature outlines how older adults tend to have visual and hearing impairments and also have issues with dexterity. Simply put, they cannot see or hear as well as they used to, and they also lack the full control of motor functions that allow for easy, fluid movements of the hand. These issues make it difficult not only to use technology but also to be able to successfully learn in the classroom. Although mental ability remains an important component of learning in old age, noncognitive factors such as visual impairment or hearing loss can decrease the efficiency with which older adults learn. In summary—if older adults cannot read a manual, or successfully maneuver a mouse, or hear an instructor, they are less likely to acquire the knowledge they need from a technology training intervention and are more likely to abandon the endeavor entirely.

The recommendations for technology instructors regarding these impairments listed below are based on previous technology intervention studies and were successfully used in our own study (these were also mentioned in the previous chapter but are worth repeating here due to their importance in understanding older students):

- Provide the *necessary tools in the technology* being taught that allow those with visual impairment to see what they are doing (whether on a screen, keypad, or so on).
- Provide *accommodations in the classroom for those who may not be able to see the instructor or to see the projected screen,* either by placing these individuals in the front of the class or providing an assistant to give one-on-one assistance.
- For those with dexterity issues or those with tremors, provide assistive devices that can help overcome these issues or opt for devices that minimize the need for motor control (e.g., using touchscreen computers rather than relying on a mouse may help with some of these issues).
- Likewise, provide *accommodations for those with hearing impairments—* again, seat these individuals in the front of the class or by a speaker, or provide one-on-one assistance.
- For the instructor, *speak loudly and slowly* when presenting material, and consider *using a microphone* when presenting

The considerations of this section and the previous one not only can improve the safety of the classroom (e.g., creating wide aisles for walking may minimize accidents as residents make their way to their workspaces) but also can help develop a rapport between the teaching staff and the residents and increase the residents' confidence in being able to successfully learn the technology and related material. Many older adults are hesitant about using a new technology simply because they feel they are too old to learn, and these feelings can be exacerbated among those with physical limitations—they may feel that they cannot learn because *they physically cannot see a screen, hear an instructor, use the technology, or even easily get to class.* Accommodating for physical limitations puts learners at ease, improves their confidence in being able to successfully complete the class, and allows them to focus their efforts on the class lessons themselves.

4.1.3 *Cognitive ability*

Although older adults have the ability to acquire and implement new knowledge similar to that of younger adults, aging can contribute to a slower and less efficient ability in information processing (Boulton-Lewis, 2010). Simply put, for many older adults it takes some extra time and practice to fully understand a new concept or to master a new activity. This can be exacerbated among older adults in a CCRC, as many have cognitive declines that inhibit their memory and prevent them from easily memorizing new material.

Information repetition is a valuable method to compensate for slower information processing. We found that repetition worked tremendously well for many of our participants learning to use a computer. In our study, repetition of content was implemented throughout the interventions in various forms:

- *Immediate repetition of new tasks.* Any time a new concept or new online activity was introduced to the class, the concept or activity was reviewed or repeated almost immediately after the initial introduction. As an example, we would have a class session devoted to opening email attachments (typically in the form of pictures); in this class, after initially showing the students how to open one attachment, we would immediately go back into their email accounts and repeat the procedures with a different attachment or a different email.

- *Reviews at the end of class.* At the end of each class session, the instructor would review all that was covered in that session, outlining any new concepts that were introduced and summarizing the different activities that were done on the devices. Not only did this remind the students of all that was done over the past 90 minutes, but also helped instill a sense of accomplishment with the residents (as many would not realize just how much new material they had learned until the end of class when it was listed for them).

- *Constant recall from previous classes (scaffolding).* Our study was structured such that each new class was built upon one of the previous sessions (e.g., the "opening email attachments class" would come after "how to open or write an email" class). Whenever this was the case, time was devoted to reviewing the material from the previous class sessions so that students were comfortable with the previous material enough to then go to the next step. After all, students new to email will not be comfortable with opening an attachment if they have not gotten a handle on opening their account and opening an email first.

- *Quizzing the students.* By quizzing, we do not mean to imply that during the classes we would hand out pieces of paper with questions on them and grade them! However, during the class sessions, we made it a habit to "quiz" the class by asking questions about previous material. As an example, on the first day of our trainings, we would always begin with showing the participants how to turn on their laptops; on the second day, rather than immediately remind the students how to turn on the laptops, we would ask the class if anyone knew or if anyone remembered how to do so from the previous session. This motivates class participation and also helps instill a sense of pride and accomplishment to those who are able to correctly answer, and it also provides a repetition of content for those who may not have memorized the material when they were initially taught it.

There may be other methods of including repetition into your training sessions to help circumvent cognitive declines that lead to slower processing speeds or slower ability at understanding new material, and the more creative you are with including it, the more fun your participants may have (and the less noticeable the repetition may be).

4.2   Organizing the environment

There is no ideal physical classroom structure that is applicable to all groups. As an example, if a class syllabus involves students working in cooperative groups to accomplish a task, then it may be wise to group students at the same table. For advanced instruction, it may behoove the class to promote increased interaction between the students and instructors (such as having the instructor seated at a table with the students).

In the context of a CCRC technology class, it is likely that you will opt for a more traditional layout, as this tends to be a successful layout when working with a large group of students who are all learning the material for the first time and do not necessarily need to interact with everyone in the class. In this section, we highlight some basic considerations when organizing an ideal classroom environment for a technology class as well as discuss how scheduling can be an important factor when finding and organizing the said environment.

4.2.1   Physical layout of the classroom

Traditional classroom arrangements typically have the students and their work areas lined up such that they are all facing one central location, such as one wall at the head of the class where a chalkboard or whiteboard and instructor are located. Common sense would dictate that a technology intervention would have a similar arrangement: rows of tables or desks with computer equipment lined up such that all are facing a wall or projection screen where an instructor's computer screen is projected for the class to see. However, such an arrangement is not always easy and is, in rare cases, impossible to achieve given the limitations of the space used as well as the needs of the residents. In this section, we outline some of the difficulties technology trainers may face when preparing a location for a technology class.

Although a stationary computer lab would be optimal for the purposes of a technology class (i.e., desktop, laptop, or tablet computers placed on desks and tables in a permanent location that is only used for technology purposes), such labs are not usually available to the residents of a CCRC. Or, if they are, they may have only a couple of computers and thus not be large enough to accommodate a group training session. Technology classes, therefore, may often be held in rooms that are designated for other purposes. In our project, we routinely had to set up our mobile computer lab in common areas, libraries, activities rooms, and even dining halls—*none of which were necessarily originally designed to accommodate a technology training session.* We had to make do with the best that was available.

Each room that is selected to house a technology class is unique in shape and in the amount of space available. Some rooms may be incredibly large and open, in which case it is relatively simple to set up rows of tables and chairs facing a projection screen. Other rooms, however, may be wide but not deep, or they may be deep but not wide (as is the case shown in Figure 4.1). Some rooms may have pillars that can block the

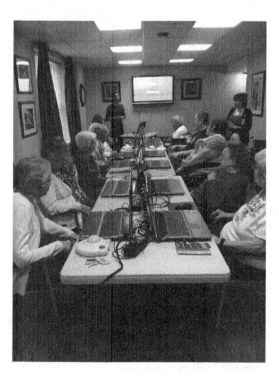

Figure 4.1 Example of a room setup in a small activities space.

students from seeing the instructor's screen. Very few spaces will afford technology instructors the perfect size and configuration that will fit all equipment and all students, and as such it may require those implementing the training to be creative with room arrangement. If rows of desks or tables are not possible, having the desks or tables arranged perpendicular to the front of the room may be ideal (as is the case shown in Figure 4.1). Tables can also be set up in various arrangements so as to maximize the amount of space used while not crowding the room (e.g., in one location we arranged tables in a horseshoe shape). Unfortunately, there is no list of perfect setup arrangements, simply because all spaces are different. Prior to a training session, instructors should take plenty of time to experiment with various room arrangements that best use the available space. Instructors should keep in mind the following points:

- How close or far away are the desks or tables from the front of the room? If students are too far away, they will not be able to see the instructor's projected screen.
- Is there enough furniture to accommodate all students (or is there too much furniture that needs to be moved so that students may more easily navigate between desks or tables)?
- The lighting in the room may not be optimal. If there is too much lighting, there may be a glare on the computer screens; if there is too little, the participants may strain to see.
- Must students have to turn their heads for an extended period of time to see the front of the room? This can be uncomfortable.

4.2.2   Scheduling: "You don't mess with bingo"

Although older adults living in CCRCs may be physically and cognitively limited in the types of activities they can do through the course of a day, many residents are still able to participate in a number of different activities, and most CCRCs have bustling activity calendars filled with such programs as exercise, musical sing-alongs, religious services, wine tastings, and games such as—yes—bingo. CCRC residents typically adhere to these schedules pretty closely as the regularity of a routine gives stability and makes the day-to-day activities more manageable. It also gives many of the residents something to look forward to when they are aware of the activities being offered and if there is something they find interesting or fun on the calendar. What we found in our study was that scheduling the technology training was not always an easy task; regardless of the residents' excitement about the training sessions, it was made clear in multiple CCRCs that residents did not want the technology trainings to interfere with their routines and with their most popular activities.

It is from this experience that we came up with the phrase "you don't mess with bingo" when arranging times for the technology training sessions (a phrase first introduced in Chapter 3). The phrase is a quote from an activity director whom we were working with when scheduling technology training. We were having difficulty identifying a time during the week where we could come in, set up the devices, conduct a 90-minute class, and take down and pack up the equipment without conflicting with another activity. When we suggested that we could potentially have the technology class overlap with a bingo session (as we had assumed bingo was an activity that a resident could show up late to or leave early from without major consequence), the activity director quickly replied with a resounding "no": if we scheduled the class against bingo, nobody would come to the class.

Mealtimes were also an important activity that many residents planned their entire days around, and in some cases, we not only had to schedule around the meals but also around the "recovery time" of the meals. In some cases, residents did not necessarily want to go straight from a meal to an activity (such as technology class) but rather wanted a bit of time to "let their food settle" before doing something else. Because of this, sometimes training sessions needed to be scheduled well after a meal was completed or, rather than being after a meal, scheduled immediately beforehand (which provided its own set of difficulties if the space being used for the class was also a dining location, as the classroom would have to quickly be converted back into a dining room before diners arrived). It will be important for the technology trainers to have an open dialogue with the staff of the CCRC, the activity director, and with the residents themselves with regard to scheduling. Carving out a time slot that does not conflict with important routines or popular activities can help maximize attendance and improve overall satisfaction with the class. Most important of all: you don't mess with bingo!

4.3   Ensuring the proper equipment

The importance of having the proper equipment was touched upon in the previous chapter. As a review, for our training we used a mobile computer lab (consisting of laptops) to teach the ICT classes, and we also made available to residents a variety of different mice and keyboards (see Table 3.2 for a complete list). It is essential to have not only enough equipment for all the residents to conduct these classes, but also backups in case something malfunctions or breaks.

There is a term used among technology researchers, introduced earlier in this book, that refers to inequalities in access to and successful use of ICTs, called the "digital divide." Whereas many technology teachers most likely concern themselves with issues involving the "second-level digital divide" (which refers to inequalities in skill and differences in attitudes toward ICTs), access to technologies can still pose a significant problem to older adults, particularly in CCRCs. In many of the CCRCs where the team went to conduct a technology training, there were very few working computers set up in common areas for the residents to use at their leisure; in some cases, the CCRC would in fact have no computers set up for the residents at all (i.e., if the residents wanted to be online, they would need to use their own devices). The computers that *were* set up were often very old and poorly maintained and also lacked assistive devices (e.g., large trackball mice and large-key keyboards) that would improve the usability of the computer for those with physical limitations. Therefore, for many of the residents, the only time they were able to use a computer and to practice the skills they learned in class was during class or during office hours; they were unable to practice on their own until we set up computers in each of the communities (discussed below).

Getting older adults online so that they may reap the potential benefits can be successfully accomplished through the implementation of a technology class or intervention, but the class will do no good if the residents have no device that they can use when the class is complete. Although it is possible that residents can purchase their own devices (as was the case with some of our participants), not all CCRC residents can afford such a purchase, and even if they can, new technology users oftentimes do not know the types of things to look for when making a computer or other ICT purchase. Therefore, to assure that CCRC technology class participants may continue to successfully use the technology after the class has been completed, access must be granted to desktop computers, laptops, or tablets and any assistive technology that the residents may require.

In our training, we would donate one desktop computer per every five study participants who completed the class and would install these computers in common areas (such as a library or a designated computer lab) for all to use. The number of computers needed per CCRC will vary based on the size of the community and the number of interested residents; however, our "one per five computer class participants" may be a good starting point. As an example, if you have a computer class and there are 20 residents who complete the class, installing four computers in common areas will likely be enough to accommodate those students (as well as other residents who want to use computers but may not have taken the class). It is also important that these computers are equipped with any assistive devices that were used in the class (e.g., special mice or keyboards).

Equipment needs go beyond having the proper technology and assistive devices for the class and for use outside the class; training staff must also plan ahead of time to have the necessary teaching equipment. Listed below are some equipment items that were used in our training sessions that may be of use in most technology trainings; again, these were elaborated upon in the previous chapter but are listed again here for reference:

- *Projector and screen.* The easiest way to teach a large group of people how to use a computer is to have an instructor's computer connected to a projector that displays the instructor's computer on a large screen. Although some CCRCs may have projectors and screens on hand, technology trainers may have to provide this equipment themselves; it is important to make this determination *before* the classes are set to begin, as you do not want to show up on the first day of class only to find out that you have no means of displaying the instructor's computer.

- *Power supplies.* You must have enough power not only for the instructor and all class participants, but also extra in case something malfunctions or breaks, or a battery loses all of its charge. In the previous chapter, we also outlined the need for many technology devices to be plugged in (either to charge or to work at all); thus, if a room configuration prevents you from stationing all devices close to a power outlet, it will be necessary to have extension cords and power strips available. Again, if possible, make this determination *before* your classes begin.

- *Training manuals.* Have enough not only for those who are beginning the technology classes, but also extra for (1) participants who accidentally lose or misplace their manuals, (2) those who decide to participate in the class *after* the first class session has already been completed (we had a few people join the class at the second or third session), and (3) those who are interested in "sitting in" or interested in learning about technology without taking the class. This was rare, but we had a couple of people who wanted to learn about computers and the Internet but could not participate in the class for one reason or another, and asked us for a manual, so they could try to teach themselves on their own. As we had extra manuals, we would always oblige.

- *Workspace furniture.* As mentioned in a previous section, not all tables and chairs will be usable for CCRC residents. Some may require chairs with a high back for support or more cushioning (or no chair at all if they are in a wheelchair), and some may require a higher table in order to fit a motorized wheelchair underneath. These are not always readily available and may require you to find these things stored somewhere at the CCRC. Although it may be difficult to determine what furniture is needed before the class begins (and you have a general sense of who is there and what they need), you should have at least a general awareness prior to starting regarding what furniture you may need to retrieve at some point. At the very least, technology trainers should know where to get these materials when needed.

The above list is not exhaustive; based on the focus of your training sessions and the subjects covered, you may be required to have additional materials. Prior to the start of training, it is crucial to outline the types of equipment and materials needed for successful implementation, and how much will be needed to accommodate the class (with extras, of course).

4.4   Designing and presenting the content

It is beyond the purview of this chapter to dictate exactly what lessons should be included in a technology class, as this will differ depending on the goals of the training, what the CCRC residents are most interested in, and what the trainers are most knowledgeable about or most comfortable with providing instruction in. As an example, because our study had a specialized research focus on social capital, the training sessions incorporated a number of lessons that taught residents to use and understand the more social aspects of the Internet, such as being able to use email to communicate with friends and family or using Facebook to connect with grandchildren or reconnect with old high school friends. At each CCRC, the staff and residents may have different ideas on what they want to cover. If you are teaching an Internet class, do you cover email and Internet searches? Do you cover social networking sites such as Facebook or cover entertainment websites like YouTube? Do you teach participants about online banking or how to find the weather report for the day? Or do you try to cover all of it? At each CCRC, the staff and residents may have different ideas on what they want to cover. Creating a comprehensive training protocol should involve a detailed discussion between those implementing the sessions and those who are attending them.

The content that is included in a lesson will also be dictated by what technology is being taught or by the devices being used; as an example, whereas it may be advantageous to teach participants how to look up the weather on the Internet if you are teaching a computer class, if you are teaching a class on smartphone use, it is more likely that the phones being used will have a weather app, and so Internet navigation will not need to be included in those lessons. There is a lot of variability with regard to what you can include in your classes, and so we have refrained from making specific content recommendations.

4.4.1   To lecture or not to lecture

Although we have refrained from listing the exact lessons one should include in a technology class, we do make recommendations on *how* the material is presented. A mixture of lecture-based classes and more inter-active classes may entice a variety of residents to participate (the lecture classes attract those who wish for more informative sessions, whereas the interactive sessions attract those who wish to have a bit of fun and hands-on experience). In our experience, the lecture-based classes were best used for lessons that students were interested in *learning* about but not neces-sarily *using* in everyday practice. As an example, we found in our training sessions that many students wanted to *learn* about Twitter, what a "tweet" was, and what it meant to "follow" someone on Twitter (as these were terms they heard on television) but very few actually wanted to open an account and *use* Twitter. In this way, we would structure the "Twitter" lesson as a traditional lecture and tell participants that if they wished to learn more and actually open an account that they should come to office hours to do so. After the class, they would be able to hold discussions with friends and family on the topic of Twitter without actually having to use the application.

Please note that this is simply an example from our study; as stated previously, the content of technology training will change from class to class, and even though our group was less interested in Twitter, your classes may be filled with students who want more hands-on train-ing with the website. In that case, it may be important to have a Twitter class be a bit more interactive: have participants create Twitter accounts, instruct them on how to search for and follow people, and teach them how to construct and post a tweet. Designing content and presentation will thus vary, again, based on the wants and needs of your class.

Another aspect that will vary between training groups is the number of class sessions being held per week and their duration. Frequency of sessions may be dictated by the schedule of the CCRC (expanded upon later in this chapter), but as for length of training sessions, we found that 90 minutes seemed to be an appropriate amount of time for the class sessions. They were long enough to cover quite a bit of material but not so long that the residents would become bored or uncomfortable. Physical discomfort can be an especially important consideration for CCRC resi-dents, as many experience quite a bit of pain when seated for long periods in uncomfortable positions.

4.4.2   Taking the content home

As stated in the previous chapter, our study involved the creation of a custom training manual that included step-by-step instruction on how to accomplish all tasks done in the class. We bring up the importance of the training manual again here because for many of our participants, the training manual was the only source of technical support they had beyond the class (other than calling us or waiting to ask questions at the next class or office hours session). A poorly designed manual that is missing lessons or lacks detailed instructions (or lacks easy-to-follow diagrams) can prevent participants from being able to review what they learn and to practice the material on their own. Creating a custom manual can be time-intensive and tiresome, and this can be exacerbated if the manual has to constantly be updated as the technology being taught is updated. However, it will ensure that your participants get the most out of their classes and can apply the lessons once formal instruction is complete.

It is possible to opt for a prepublished technology training manual, but it may not cover all the lessons being covered, may not be written specifically for older adults with little to no technology experience, or may cover topics the residents may deem uninteresting. We typically received rave reviews from participants in our study, mostly because the manual mirrored the in-class instructions almost verbatim; they found that when they were sitting at a computer by themselves outside of class, looking at the manual was almost comparable to having the instructor there with them. Therefore, we caution that if you are opting to use a prepublished training manual to cut down on time and labor, try to find a manual that mirrors your lessons or adjust your lessons so that how the material is presented in class is comparable to how it is presented in the manual. This will make out-of-class practice easier and less confusing for participants.

Tips for designing an effective training manual suggested by most educational gerontologists include the following:

- Use easy-to-identify headings to group the content into well-organized sections
- Use boldface type or underlining for headings or to identify important concepts (italic type tends to be more difficult to read for those with visual impairment)
- Create gaps in the text between sections so that participants may more easily see the beginning of a new section (this also helps participants organize the content in their minds)
- Repeat important concepts frequently and summarize your main points at the end of each section
- Include screen shots to illustrate how to complete tasks, identify parts of devices, and so on
- Use easy-to-see pictures, tables, and diagrams

4.5 Engaging and motivating participants

We have discussed the learning needs of CCRC populations, how to structure the learning environment, the necessary equipment, and the content of the classes. What comes next, on paper, may seem like the easiest thing a trainer can do as it seems less labor-intensive: motivating and engaging older adults in the classroom. However, keeping older learners motivated to continue attending classes even when they experience difficulties with the material or lack confidence in their ability to continue can be a challenge. In this section, we outline ways in which technology trainers can keep their students coming back to class: making sure instructors are sociable and well-versed in the material, assembling a positive assistive team, instilling a "practice makes perfect" mantra, and promoting a community within the CCRC wherein residents help one another when difficulties with the technology arise.

4.5.1 Training the trainer

Recommending that the instructors of a technology intervention be well-versed and knowledgeable in the technologies they are teaching and the online practices they are demonstrating seems obvious. After all, how would students learn anything from a chemistry professor who did not understand molecules, or how would athletes learn how to swim properly from a coach who had never been in water before? But when we make the recommendation to "train the trainer," we are not simply insisting that the trainers themselves be experts on the topics being covered; we are also implying that the trainers need to be instructed on *how to best present these topics specifically to a class with older adults in CCRCs.*

This is easier said than done, as presenting information to a crowd of older CCRC residents can be vastly different from presenting information to a typical classroom of students. Instructors must be sure to enunciate clearly and substantially increase the volume of their voices not only so that those in the back of the class can hear but also so that those who are hard of hearing have an easier time listening and understanding. Instructors must also speak more slowly than they may usually be accustomed to, as this allows older adults with slower cognitive processing speed to better absorb the material. Having an instructor who is constantly repeating statements and recalling earlier topics can also help those with slower cognitive processing to absorb the lessons. This is not always a simple task, as some instructors may find the constant repetition of material to be tedious and boring (and if the instructor is bored, the students will know it). A bit of patience with students and the material can go a long way to assure that the residents learning the technology get the most out of the class and enjoy the experience.

Finally, while it may be difficult to "teach" a trainer on the attitudes best displayed in a training situation, a trainer can at least be cognizant of the types of attitudes older adults in CCRCs respond positively to. In the case of our training sessions, participants responded best to an attitude of friendly professionalism wherein the instructors demonstrated a confident command of the material but did not refrain from being sociable with the participants. ALC and ILC residents tend to enjoy sharing personal stories and enjoy getting to know their instructors, and thus training a trainer to be social (while maintaining a bit of authority like any other teacher) can make the sessions more fun for participants.

4.5.2 *The importance of a supportive teaching team*

Although the lead instructor of a technology training will no doubt be the center of attention during the class sessions, a lone instructor may find it difficult to accomplish all the tasks necessary for a successful training session, including coordinating a time and place for the classes, classroom setup, lesson preparation, fielding questions from students, cleaning up, and so on. Having a team in place that is supportive of one another can lead to a more efficient technology class wherein the strains on the lead instructor are minimized and the instructor may more thoroughly concentrate his or her efforts on the lessons themselves.

When we recommend that a teaching team be "supportive," we do not restrict this definition to "a team that is supportive of one another." We also define it as a team that is supportive of the students. Learning anything new, including something as complicated as using a new technology, can be overwhelming for older adults in CCRCs, especially if they have experienced cognitive declines that impede the learning process and make it difficult to absorb information. Frustrations can easily mount, but having a training staff that is constantly assisting the residents and constantly encouraging them can go a long way to improving the confidence of the students. In our training sessions, we would have the teaching team walk around the room during class and keep an eye on all participants, addressing any questions that were asked and identifying participants who may be struggling but were wary of directly asking for help; in addition, the teaching team would speak directly to the students about their progress and accomplishments, highlighting the amount of material they covered and how much success they had in the day. Even small, almost innocuous, bits of encouragement can be enough motivation for the students to continue with the lessons and strive for success, and it may put them at ease to know that they have a teaching team that is there to not only provide technical support but also emotional support as well.

4.5.3 Practice makes perfect

Although feedback for the technology classes we implemented trended toward positive comments, frustration was commonplace among some of the students of our study, particularly for those suffering from slight cognitive decline or slight memory issues. The frustrations voiced by residents, however, were less focused on the instructors and classes and instead more on the disappointment in their own abilities. The following quote was taken from a focus group session and exemplifies thoughts by residents at other CCRCs:

> *Presider*: Do you think you will need more training to be able to maintain your current level of usage? Why or why not?
> *Ms. M.*: I feel stupid. We expect first graders to read after a few weeks and…I just don't feel I've learned as much as I could have.

Speaking broadly about the "digital divide" and digital inequality, Millward (2003) argues that difficulties in learning to use ICTs may contribute to feelings of disappointment, embarrassment, and humiliation, and may in fact motivate individuals to stop using the technology altogether. Millward (2003) states that "If some individuals have tried and failed to use [the] Internet, they are more likely to say that they have 'no interest' in doing so, rather than reporting their actual lack of skills."

Thus, constant encouragement is recommended for CCRC residents trying to learn to use a computer and the Internet. In our experience, whenever an individual voiced frustration with their inability to use the technology or difficulties in recalling items that were taught in class, a way to help alleviate the frustration was to tell the students that computers are complicated and take a quite a bit of time and (above all else) practice to master. Oftentimes, we would share with the participants our own frustrations with learning to use a new program or a new device, usually revealing by the end that the only way we became comfortable with the technology was through constant use. We would also relay the experiences of others like them, older adults with little to no computer experience who through time, patience, and practice managed to master the technology. Sharing the success stories of others illustrated that inexperience and difficulties in the learning process do not necessarily dictate whether the person will be able to use the technology, and that determination and perseverance can go a long way. By telling the students that they are not alone in their frustrations and that these frustrations can be overcome with patience and practice, students are more likely to stick with the class and work through the difficulties they may encounter.

4.5.4   Ask your neighbor—promoting a community where residents help one another

Although participants of our study benefitted from frequent interaction with instructors and training personnel both in the classroom and during the optional office hours sessions, educational and technical support were limited to the period of time in which the study was conducted; once the study was complete, the instructors and training personnel would no longer be available to the participants to assist with the technologies and to answer inquiries on their use. This raised the question: How would the participants receive assistance should they encounter difficulties with the technologies? Who would be on hand to answer detailed inquiries about using the technologies or to demonstrate how to use applications that were not covered in the class sessions or the training manual? One of the methods by which the training personnel sought to overcome this potential issue was to promote a community in which the residents themselves acted as instructors and assisted one another should computer and Internet questions arise (see Figure 4.2).

With regard to technology training, peer teaching/learning models have shown to be as effective in promoting use of ICTs and in promoting confidence in use as have more traditional instructor-directed models (Woodward et al., 2013). Older learners argue that trainers who are older tend to have similar life experiences and thus better understand the physical and psychosocial needs of the student as well as specific

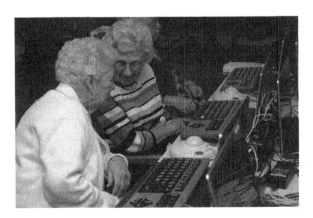

Figure 4.2 Intervention participant asks her neighbor for assistance.

interests, and the process of learning from someone of a similar age can be more fun and enjoyable as a result (Xie, 2007). Our team thought it would thus be advantageous to promote a community in which the study participants could help one another once the study was complete and the instructors and training personnel were no longer available. To create a successful peer-learning environment, two strategies were implemented: (1) identifying "resident experts" who showed increased ICT understanding and could serve as a tutor for struggling residents and (2) promoting a social atmosphere in which residents were unafraid to engage with one another when using ICTs.

Identifying a resident expert typically occurred over the course of the technology training. If one of the residents showed increased knowledge and competence in using ICTs, he or she was asked by the study team if he or she would feel comfortable serving as tutor once the study was complete. These experts were often, but not always, individuals who had computer and Internet experience prior to the class. When proposing this to the potential expert, the study team often highlighted how serving as an expert could double as a form of community service and "giving back" to the other residents. In most cases, the expert would have no issue with serving as an expert unless he or she lacked confidence in his or her own abilities. Depending on the size of the class, it was sometimes necessary to appoint multiple experts.

Promoting a social atmosphere occurred both during the classes and during office hours. When possible, the study team would attempt to identify individuals taking the class who had previous computer and Internet experience early in the class or even prior to the class, during the screening and baseline survey stage. Using this knowledge, the study team would attempt to manipulate the seating chart such that those with computer and Internet experience were interspersed throughout the classroom. This would sometimes be difficult, as many residents would have specific requests as to where they would like to be seated during class, but it was possible. By spacing out those with computer experience, it gave inexperienced participants easy access to individuals who might be able to provide assistance should the instructors and training personnel be unavailable. During the classes and during office hours, the study team would encourage the residents to speak with one another, share their triumphs and difficulties during the class, and work together to overcome obstacles. In this way, residents would, over time, become comfortable with one another and rely on one another to solve simple or complex computer or Internet issues rather than rely solely on the study team and their manuals. Creating a community where residents can assist one another can provide a safety net in situations where the training staff are not always or readily available. Also, in situations where training staff are available 24/7, creating an atmosphere such as this may lift some of the time and effort burden off of the staff.

4.6 Other considerations

In addition to the complexities highlighted previously in this chapter, there are a few other things technology trainers need to take into consideration when designing a class for older adults. We highlight three of them here: using activity directors to your advantage, enabling older learners to adapt to new technologies, and accounting for attrition.

4.6.1 The importance of engaged activity directors

In addition to having a supportive teaching team, having a supportive and engaged activity director can also help in fostering a comfortable and enjoyable learning environment at the CCRCs. Of all the individuals who work at a CCRC, the employee that residents are most likely to see the most often (besides perhaps the dining staff) is the activity director (who sometimes has the title of activities coordinator or something similar). With many CCRCs having an activity calendar filled to the brim with such things as games, music, and trips, an active older adult living in a CCRC would likely see the activity director multiple times during the day as he or she attended the variety of activities offered. Because of these interactions, many activity directors already have a strong rapport with the residents, and technology teachers would be wise to utilize this relationship to their advantage. Some of the ways in which the activity director was able to meaningfully contribute to our training sessions included the following:

- *Recruitment.* Although we would have our own recruitment session at the CCRCs to try to get people to sign up for our technology classes, in many instances, we would get additional sign-ups from the hard work of activity directors who would knock on the doors of residents to tell them about the classes, post flyers throughout the CCRCs, and announce the coming of the classes at other activities. Also, because the activity director is typically someone who is well-liked and appreciated among the residents, individuals who were "on the fence" with regard to participating in the class would often opt into signing up after hearing about the classes from the activity director (someone they know and trust rather than a stranger).
- *Relationships with other CCRC staff.* The most salient example of this for us involved the need for additional assistance with the setup. At many of the CCRCs where we held technology classes, the space

we used for the classes did not have enough furniture to hold all of the computers; we needed additional tables and chairs. The activity director would oftentimes be the point of contact between us and the housing/maintenance staff who had access to additional tables and chairs, as the activity directors themselves would oftentimes need to get in contact with housing/maintenance for their own planned activities. Therefore, by developing a relationship with the activity director, you are also injecting yourself into a network of CCRC staff that can assist with the technology classes.

- *Setup and takedown.* An extra body is an extra body, and having the activity director there to assist with the setup of a mobile lab and packing it up at the end can help save time; however, it is important to train the activity director the proper way to accomplish both of these tasks (as, in our case, we had numerous instances where an activity director would improperly pack up computer equipment and we would have to repack it so that everything would fit correctly into storage).
- *Class excitement and motivation.* As stated previously, activity directors can lead the list of CCRC staff the residents see most often and thus trust the most. Therefore, having the activity director at the technology classes themselves can help foster a strong relationship between the teaching staff and the students. Having a trustworthy individual in the class environment to help the residents, answer questions, and (if need be) "vouch" for the teaching staff can put participants at ease. It can also increase excitement among students (because they will have someone they know and like there with them) and thus increase motivation to stay and learn.

Unfortunately, not every CCRC will have a particularly popular or particularly engaged activity director who is willing to assist with the classes or is able to provide additional support. In our experience, however, having an unpopular or disliked activity director is unusual, as these individuals tended to be the ones residents cited the most often as the most helpful and fun. More often than not, the activity director can prove to be a vital asset who can bridge the relationship between the teaching staff and CCRC staff or the teaching staff and the residents themselves.

4.6.2   Enabling the older adult to adapt to rapidly changing technology

During one of the last training sessions of our ICT study, a CCRC resident came up to the training staff regarding her new laptop. It had been given to her as a gift and she was wondering if she could bring it to one of the optional office hours sessions for assistance in learning to navigate the interface. The study team told her that it was fine and that we had had countless other residents do the same thing: bring their own devices to office hours so that they could practice the lessons on equipment they would be using in their homes.

Even though the computers we used in the classes typically had many of the same attributes as the residents' personal devices, small differences between the technologies could sometimes reveal themselves as huge hurdles to the residents' understanding of technology. Things seemingly as innocuous as having a different default homepage upon opening an Internet browser could cause confusion and frustration, especially to those who had never used the technology before and were relying solely on the exact things learned in class; if an icon or background looked different from what was presented in class, or if something was located in a different place on the screen from where the resident was used to, it could be enough for them to give up completely.

It can be difficult to give older adults in CCRCs the necessary tools that enable them to adapt to rapidly evolving technologies, as it is difficult to predict exactly *how* technology is going to change over time. As an example, who knew a decade ago that tablet computers with touchscreen interfaces would not only be available to the public but would also be incredibly popular and affordable, such that millions of people would use them? Therefore, technology trainers need to be up-to-date on the latest devices, applications, and websites so that they can be taught to CCRC residents without fear of the residents being "behind the times" and thus unable to use the technology.

It is also important to assist the residents in mastering the basics of using a technology such that, should the technology change, the residents will at least have a starting point in which to experiment from and try to figure out (i.e., learn) the evolved technology. As an example, teaching the residents that a "gear" symbol in a webpage usually signifies a help menu or a settings menu can provide them with a visual reference if they go to their email inbox only to find that the layout has changed inexplicably (as was actually the case during our training sessions, as in one class where the layouts of all our participants' inboxes became updated and visually changed, confusing the residents). No trainer will be able to account for everything, as it is impossible to predict how technology will change, and so making sure that the residents have a technical support network (whether in the form of an onsite information technology expert or motivating the residents to have a computer club) can also prove vital.

Of special note is that technology trainers not only will need to account for updated technologies in their class sessions but also must account for them in their training materials, such as a computer manual. Whether it is because a visual layout is updated, a program or application has added features, or a technology has a new operating system, training manuals need to be updated so that CCRC residents are not confused when using this reference to troubleshoot or to practice their skills. Keeping an updated manual can prove to be excruciatingly tedious work as it may require the constant changing of instructions and picture aids, and it can be made even more difficult if the technology being taught is updated on a regular basis. However, having updated training materials is a necessity to assure student success.

4.6.3   Expecting attrition

As with any other intervention or training activities, technology interventions are susceptible to high attrition rates, or an elevated level of dropouts. Any intervention involving older adults is particularly susceptible to increased attrition rates due to a number of factors; a review of longitudinal studies conducted by Bhamra and colleagues (Bhamra et al., 2008) found that being older, being more cognitively impaired, having less education, having a lower socioeconomic status, being less socially active, and having worse health are all risk factors for attrition in older adult populations. In our study, we experienced firsthand the difficulties associated with dropouts. Although we were able to initially recruit 324 participants for the study (314 of which passed our cognitive screening instrument), only 256 participants completed the preintervention and postintervention assessment, and only 208 completed all follow-up assessments (as a reminder, our study went on for a full year after the interventions were completed). For our study, the most cited reasons for participant dropout were health concerns, lack of participation, relocation, loss of interest, and death.

Unfortunately, training personnel may not be able to address all the particular reasons why an older adult in a CCRC chooses to withdraw from a technology class. Little can be done if a participant becomes sick and cannot attend technology class or if a participant decides to move away from the CCRC. But although the technology trainers may not be able to account for all possible reasons for attrition, some—like loss of interest—can be prevented by keeping the technology interventions interactive and enjoyable and by keeping the participants engaged throughout. We found that our participants tended to remain interested in the classes if they found the lessons to be applicable to their wants and needs; as an example, our original training plan included equal time spent on teaching email and social media, but as the study progressed and we found participants were much more interested in email than social media, we increased the time spent teaching email and reduced the hours spent on teaching about sites like Facebook and Twitter.

Participants remained more engaged when they were asked to participate in the lesson as well; as an example, when teaching the participants about searching for information online, we would ask the class for suggestions on "what to Google." Something as simple as asking for a search topic can go a long way in keeping the participants engaged with the instructors and engaged with the material (and when asking the class for topics to search, you can get varied responses that may inject a bit of humor into the proceedings). Finally, keeping things light and fun also assisted in battling disinterest; as an example, when teaching participants how to open email attachments, we would send them emails with either humorous pictures with animals or pictures of local landmarks to open.

Battling disinterest can be an adaptive process for the instructors. As previously mentioned, we adapted our classes to include more email-focused sessions once we learned that the participants preferred to learn about that topic. Adaptations like this happened frequently, with us expanding some lessons and condensing or even cutting others. Unfortunately, not every class environment will be the same, and so instructors may be left with making quite a few judgment calls on which topics to cover and which to gloss over. For our project, having optional office hours (where participants could receive one-on-one instruction beyond the normal class sessions) allowed participants to learn about topics that were not covered in the class and thus any topic that was condensed or cut could still be taught to the participants. However, not every CCRC setting may be equipped to have office hours sessions like we did, and so instructors must be mindful about creating and adapting a class schedule that remains fun and engaging while also not ignoring topics CCRC residents may want covered.

4.7 Summary of best practices

Constructing and implementing a successful technology training program can require quite a bit of work, and special considerations must be made when tailoring a program to the needs of older adults living in CCRCs. Below is a list of guidelines we recommend that technology trainers follow when beginning their own training sessions in community settings; it is our hope that these guidelines will increase the likelihood that trainers will be able to conduct an efficient and smooth technology

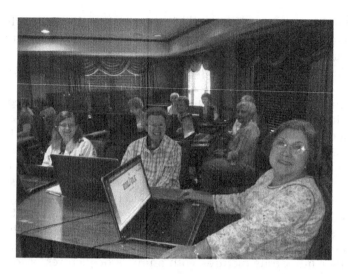

Figure 4.3 Intervention participants smiling for the camera during class.

training that participants not only will gain much out of but also will find comfortable and enjoyable (see Figure 4.3).

- *Understanding the learner.* Take into account the physical and cognitive limitations of your students. To overcome mobility issues, hold the technology class in the CCRC at a central location, and provide furniture that is comfortable for prolonged seating. Provide a means for sick individuals to makeup missed classes. Put those with visual or hearing impairments toward the front of the class, and use a microphone when teaching. Speak loudly and slowly. Provide assistive devices to accommodate those with dexterity issues. Incorporate repetition into the protocol to account for slower processing speeds and declining cognitive ability.
- *Organizing the environment.* Use a traditional classroom setup when possible if you are dealing with a large number of new students. Try to find a space that comfortably fits all students, trainers, and equipment (including tables and chairs) but also allows for mobility in the classroom (so that older adults with walkers, canes, or wheelchairs will not be inhibited in movement). Be cognizant of little details, such as how far away students are from the main projection screen, or the lighting in the room. Schedule the class so as not to overlap with other important activities, and be sure the room you are using is not only available for class but also for setup and takedown.

- *Ensuring the proper equipment.* Have enough technological devices (and backups) for all participants and trainers. Make sure there are also a projector and screen, ample power supplies, enough training manuals, and enough furniture. Provide devices in public areas for CCRC residents to use outside of class to practice what they have learned.
- *Creating and presenting content.* Listen to the residents and teach what they want to learn! If they do not want to know about Facebook, do not spend 4 weeks covering the intricacies of creating and using an account. Experiment with lecture and more interactive formats (lectures are best reserved for straightforward presentation of concepts). Take the time and effort to create a usable training manual, custom-made for your classes, that mirrors the lessons (or conversely, find a suitable prepublished manual and adapt your classes to mirror the manual).
- *Engaging and motivating participants.* Be sure that instructors are well-versed in the topics they are covering in class and be sure that they are adequately prepared to present these topics to a CCRC audience in a loud, slow voice, and with an attitude of friendly professionalism. Surround the lead instructor with a teaching team who support one another while also being supportive of the students, both in a technical and in an emotional capacity. Battle discouragement and a lack of confidence in technological abilities among participants by enforcing the notion that "practice makes perfect." Promote a community where residents will help one another in the absence of an instructor.
- *Other considerations.* Develop a strong relationship with the activity director to foster a rapport with the CCRC residents and with other CCRC staff; the activity director may also be able to supply additional assistance during the classes, if needed. Keep up with the latest technological advances and make efforts to prepare the participants, should they be exposed to these advances. Battle disinterest by engaging participants and keeping the classes light and fun.

As mentioned, the recommendations provided are based on previous studies and educational gerontology theories as well our experiences with teaching older adults in CCRCs. It needs to be stressed, though, that no two classrooms are alike, and the needs of the class will change based on a variety of factors, including the preferences of the students, the abilities of the instructors, the equipment available, and the culture of the CCRC. Thus, our best recommendation for technology instructors is this: be prepared for anything!

Recommended readings

Chaffin, A. J. and Harlow, S. D. 2005. Cognitive learning applied to older adult learners and technology. *Educational Gerontology, 31,* 301–329.

Duay, D. L. and Bryan, V. C. 2008. Learning in later life: What seniors want in a learning experience. *Educational Gerontology, 34,* 1070–1086.

Purdie, N. and Boulton-Lewis, G. 2003. The learning needs of older adults. *Educational Gerontology, 29,* 129–149.

Stevens, B. 2003. How seniors learn. *Issue Brief: Center for Medicare Education,* 4(9), 1–8.

chapter five

Value of technology training

As discussed in earlier chapters of this book, technological devices and applications have a wide variety of potential benefits to users. The obvious benefits are practical ones, as devices such as Internet-connected computers and smartphones grant users unprecedented access to information that can improve daily living, provide new methods of communication to help reinforce old relationships and social ties, and be used to develop new relationships. For example, a person with diabetes may use an Internet-connected smartphone to find information on popular and reliable treatment methods or possibly download an application (or "app") that can help treat and manage the disease. Likewise, a person with depression may use a search engine (such as Google) on any Internet-connected device to look for online treatment options and assistance in managing symptoms. With regard to communication, people with a mental health issue such as depression can access online support groups or forums and engage with others to discuss experiences and evaluate treatment options.

A successful technological intervention can improve people's ability to use devices and applications both in an information-seeking and communicative capacity; that is, a technology class can train people to better find health information online and train people to get in touch with friends, family, and others (including doctors) to discuss health considerations. But there are benefits of a technology training that go beyond just the more immediate practical considerations, as technology classes have the potential to promote more positive attitudes toward technology, increase self-efficacy (i.e., a person's belief in his or her own success), increase overall technology use, and improve quality of life. These benefits can be especially pronounced in CCRC populations, as older adults tend to have more negative attitudes toward computers and the Internet and have lower technology use compared to other age groups. CCRC residents are also at risk of feeling detached from society, less autonomous and in control of their lives, and less enriched and fulfilled. Technology use can help to mitigate these negative feelings and attitudes.

The purpose of this chapter is to discuss the potential benefits of technology training for older adults by highlighting findings from previous research studies as well as discussing specific results from our study (previously presented in depth in Chapter 3). Although the costs of implementing a technology intervention in a CCRC can be high when all things are considered (including the price of equipment, transportation, and hiring instructors), the advantages of technology training to the residents are numerous, such as connecting them with family and friends, encouraging positive attitudes toward technology, and helping them feel more connected to society. These and other benefits justify the potential expense (money, effort, *and* time) associated with the training.

5.1   Changing attitudes and self-efficacy

With all of the communication and information-sharing potential of technology, it is no wonder that there have been significant increases in the past few decades in the number of people who are using such devices as Internet-connected computers, cellphones or smartphones, and tablets. According to Perrin and Duggan (2015), older adults remain the age group that uses technologies the least, but the proportion of users continues to grow. This trend is illustrated in Figure 5.1, which shows that although the percentage of older adults in the United States who use the Internet still lags behind the general adult population (where 86% report going online), the percentage of older adults who go online has seen a very large increase between 2000 and 2015, from 14% to 58%. The growing number of older adults using technology can be taken as a sign that many older adults are conquering what has been termed the "digital divide," or the inequalities associated with access to and use of technologies, particularly information and communication technologies (ICTs).

It is the second part of this gap—the inequalities associated with *use* of technologies (rather than access)—that has been of particular interest to researchers in the past few years. In the late 1990s and early 2000s, the primary focus of those looking to explore and decrease the digital divide primarily examined differences in access between different groups; the argument was that the reason certain groups of people did not use ICTs was that they could not access them. For example, those without access might include people living in a rural area where broadband Internet connectivity was unavailable or people living in poverty who could not afford to purchase an ICT device. However, although issues of access do remain an important component of the digital divide, in the early 2000s, many researchers began to explore what came to be called a "second-level digital divide" that focuses on barriers to successful use of ICTs that go beyond issues of ownership and access; components of the second-level divide include attitudes toward technology, knowledge of and familiarity with technology, and skill level and technical expertise.

For instructors of technology classes, increasing technology knowledge and skill level is a primary goal of the class. A technology class

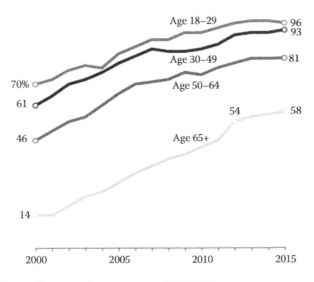

Young adults are most likely to use the Internet, but
seniors show faster adoption rates

Among all American adults, the percentage who use Internet, by age

Source: Pew research center surveys, 2000–2015.
PEW research center

Figure 5.1 Pew Research Center statistics on the percentage of older adults (age 65+) who go online compared to other age groups. (From Perrin, A., and Duggan, M., *Americans' internet access: 2000–2015*, Pew Research Center, Washington, DC, 2015. Retrieved from http://www.pewinternet.org/2015/06/26/americans-internet-access-2000-2015/)

can help decrease issues associated with the second-level digital divide by giving groups of people who are at risk for decreased technology use the tools to increase successful use of various devices and applications. However, most technology instructors may not take into consideration how a technology class may also *change classroom attitudes* both toward the technologies being taught as well as toward the class participants themselves. The remainder of this section details how attitudes toward technology and toward the self can impact technology usage (with examples from our study).

5.1.1 *Attitudes toward ICTs*

Successful use of technology by older adults can be inhibited by negative attitudes toward the technology as well as self-perceptions that the individual is unable to learn to use the technology. Negative attitudes can manifest in a variety of forms, such as feeling intimidated by the technology, finding it frustrating to learn or to use, expressing disinterest in learning or using technology, or arguing that the individual has no need to use the technology. For older adults to receive the full benefit of using technology, they must first overcome these negative attitudes. They must be convinced that there is a benefit to be gained before embarking on the sometimes arduous process of learning to use new and emerging technologies. As seen in Figure 5.2, many older adults simply do not feel they are "missing out on much."

Lack of knowledge and skill are oft-cited reasons older adults choose not to use technologies, and we observed this firsthand in our study. During many of our recruitment sessions, CCRC residents were often hesitant to sign up for the classes, fearing that they did not know enough about computers to even get started with one, would not be able to keep pace with the

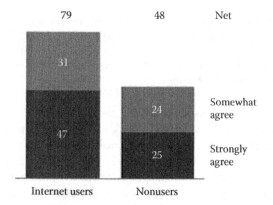

Many older noninternet users don't think they are missing out on much

Percentage of those 65 and older who agree with the statement: "People without internet access are at a real disadvantage because of all the information they might be missing"

79   48   Net

31

                          Somewhat
               24   agree

47
                          Strongly
               25   agree

Internet users   Nonusers

PEW research center's Internet project july 18–september 30, 2013 tracking survey

PEW research center

Figure 5.2 Pew Research Center statistics on attitudes toward Internet access and "missing out" on information. (From Smith, A., *Older adults and technology use*, Pew Research Center, Washington, DC, 2014. Retrieved from http://www.pewinternet.org/2014/04/03/older-adults-and-technology-use/)

others in the class, or would break the equipment after making a mistake. As discussed in Chapters 3 and 4, reassurances by the study personnel would become key in recruiting participants into the class and keeping them in the study (done by continually telling the residents that the classes were structured for beginners, that the material was repeated, that the equipment could not be easily broken, and so on). Beyond this, however, is the issue of attitudes toward technology as a potential barrier to successful use.

As part of our study, we investigated whether an 8-week technological intervention in a CCRC had a significant effect on attitudes toward computers among residents. In the surveys that were administered to the CCRC residents pre- and postintervention (i.e., before the technology classes began and after the 8 weeks of classes had concluded), we asked to what degree they agreed or disagreed with various statements that measured attitudes toward computers, examples of which include "Computers make me uncomfortable," "I feel intimidated by computers," and "Computers are difficult to understand." We analyzed whether there was any change in level of agreement or disagreement with these statements between the first survey (preintervention) and the second survey (postintervention). The results as shown in Figure 5.3 showed that a

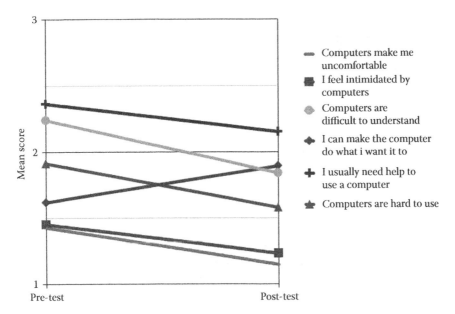

Figure 5.3 Changes in attitudes toward computers from pre- to postintervention in our study (scores ranged from 0 to 4, with higher scores indicating higher agreement with a statement). (From Berkowsky, R.W. et al. *Educational Gerontology*, 39, 797–811, 2013.)

technological intervention could lead to more positive attitudes toward technology. Residents were less likely to feel uncomfortable or intimidated, and more likely to disagree that computers are hard to use. They indicated that they felt more positively about understanding computers and about their ability to actually use a computer without assistance. They also reported a greater ability to use a computer for their own purposes.

These findings are similar to what other studies have postulated (see the Recommended Readings section at the end of this chapter)— that a technology intervention can significantly foster positive attitudes toward the technology. This is an important finding that many researchers and instructors may ignore; that is, although older adults can benefit from technology, they will be less willing to use it (and thus less likely to reap the benefits) if they consistently harbor negative attitudes. A well-designed intervention that highlights the strengths of the technology and helps older adults overcome fears, anxieties, and frustrations with the technology, can go a long way in helping users scale the second-level digital divide and use the technology to its full potential.

5.1.2   Self-efficacy

Beyond changing attitudes toward the technology, technology interventions and trainings can also help change attitudes toward the self. A popular concept in the field of psychology and an important component in social cognitive theory is that of *self-efficacy*. Bandura (1982), the conceptual developer, explained:

> Knowledge, transformational operations, and component skills are necessary but insufficient for accomplished performances. Indeed, people often do not behave optimally, even though they know full well what to do. This is because self-referent thought also mediates the relationship between knowledge and action. The issues addressed in this line of inquiry are concerned with how people judge their capabilities and how, through their self-percepts of efficacy, they affect their motivation and behavior (p. 122).

Put another way, self-efficacy can be defined as an individual's self-evaluation in the ability to achieve certain goals or how much an individual "believes in" himself or herself. Although similar to both self-esteem and confidence, self-efficacy is distinct from these constructs. Self-esteem tends to be tied to self-worth, and thus perceived ability to achieve a goal may not contribute to self-esteem if the goal is not an important one. An example is an older adult who is learning to use a new appliance, such as a new stove. If the older adult is having trouble learning to set the timer or clock, he or she may have low self-efficacy (due to a perceived inability to master the technique) but not low self-esteem (if the task of setting the clock or timer is unimportant to him or her because he or she does not really need the clock or timer). Confidence, in contrast, typically refers to the strength an individual has in believing in himself or herself but may not specifically refer to belief in accomplishing a goal (i.e., an older adult trying to use a new stove may be confident in success *or* failure). Therefore, self-efficacy incorporates aspects of both self-esteem and confidence.

A study examining how self-efficacy, computer knowledge, and computer anxiety could contribute to overall feelings of life satisfaction in older adults living in private residences in the Southern part of Florida was conducted by Karavidas, Lim, and Katsikas (2005). The results of the study indicate that technology use can positively impact self-efficacy; thus, it can be assumed that a successful technology intervention that increases technology skill would also increase self-efficacy. Indeed, studies have shown this and found a relationship between time spent online and computer self-efficacy among older adults in assisted and independent living communities who had participated in a training course to learn about computers and how to surf the Web.

Self-efficacy was not directly measured in our study survey instrument; however, the survey data suggested that the technology intervention did have a positive impact on self-efficacy. To illustrate, there was a general increase among study participants in feelings that they were able to "make the computer do what they wanted to." This can be interpreted that, with regard to computer use, participants were more confident in their ability to successfully operate a computer as a result of the training. Moreover, there was a significant change between the initial preintervention and the postintervention surveys in response to survey questions and statements regarding limitations associated with technology use. As an example, fewer participants in our study indicated that computers and the Internet were "too hard to use" after completion of the technology classes, showing that the respondents perceived fewer obstacles and could overcome barriers to use (see Figure 5.4).

In addition to the quantitative findings from our survey data, there were informative findings in our qualitative data taken from field notes, focus groups, and so on. We found numerous instances where participants verbally indicated that their belief in themselves improved over the course of the study. Whether they were new to learning how to use a computer and were starting from scratch or were experienced users who were taking the class as a way to brush up on their skills

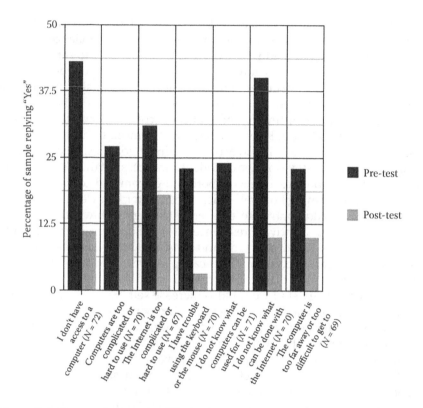

Figure 5.4 Changes in perceived limitations to using computers and the Internet. (From Berkowsky, R.W. et al. *Educational Gerontology, 39,* 797–811, 2013.)

or learn about a new procedure or application, the participants mostly came away from the interventions with a sense of accomplishment in what they had done and what they could do in the future. Comments included the following:

> You brought me into the twenty-first century. I became more knowledgeable on the computer after 11 years of having it sit there. I have shocked some people by sending [email] (Ms. T., focus group participant).

5.2 Technology use across the study

As previously discussed, issues related to the digital divide pertain to inequalities in access to and use of technologies, and older adults are an at-risk group of being on the wrong side of the divide. However, intervention studies have shown that older adults, including those who live in CCRCs, can overcome limitations associated with using a computer or the Internet and can have more positive attitudes toward technology as a result of technology training, which may in turn promote increased technology use. But although results of our study and others show that a technology intervention can increase positive attitudes toward technology, there remains a question regarding technology classes and actual use. In other words, can a technology class *actually increase technology usage* among older adults, and (if so) is this effect long term?

What we found in our study when examining trends in technology usage pre- and postintervention was that there was a significant increase in use, specifically with regard to going online and accessing and using websites (which was a particular focus of our training). However, the effects of the training on usage levels dissipated over time, as we saw when we examined the survey data taken from our participants at the 3-, 6-, and 12-month follow-up visits. This is not an unexpected occurrence (and the reasons for decreased usage after the training was complete are discussed later in this section). As shown in Figure 5.5, there were significant increases in the number of Internet-related activities between the pre- and the postintervention surveys, including going online; using email; surfing the Web; playing games alone; searching for information regarding hobbies, movies, leisure, or entertainment; visiting the websites of family and friends; checking the news and weather; and using social networking sites. There were a number of activities that saw no increase postintervention, such as shopping and using instant messaging programs. A majority of the activities where we saw change in usage were *topics that were covered in the class*, suggesting that, for most things covered in our intervention, usage successfully increased among our participants.

Of the activities for which an increase was noticed, most of the increase dissipated over the course of a year, such that activity levels returned to their preintervention baseline or close to it. However, dissipation was *not* seen for four activities: going online, using email, surfing the Web, and playing games alone (highlighted in bold in Figure 5.5). Going online, using email, and surfing the Web were covered in great detail during the intervention and were repeatedly practiced throughout the course, which led to continued use even after the intervention was complete.

The focus groups conducted at the end of the training sessions at each site shed some light as to why many individuals did not keep up a high level of usage on some activities once the training sessions were complete. A common theme among residents was that without continued technological support to answer questions for them, in the event of facing

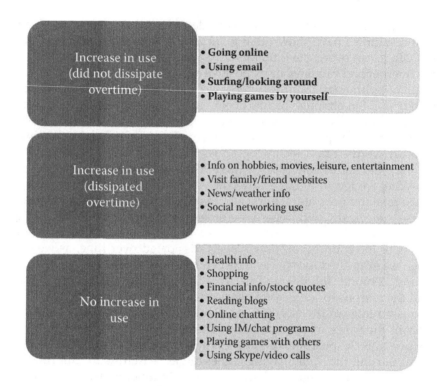

Figure 5.5 Changes in technology usage between pre- and postintervention (usage was measured as how often participants performed each task, with responses ranging from several times a week to not at all).

difficulties the residents would opt to give up rather than seek outside help to answer questions:

> I'm afraid I might have a question that you guys could clear up in a few minutes, even over the phone. Our memories are not like they used to be. Some people in here are getting old [laughs] (Mr. S., focus group participant).

There were instances where residents tried to circumvent the lack of more professional technical support by suggesting that those who participated in the technology intervention create an informal "computer club" that could meet and use the computer together. In this way, if anyone ran into any trouble while using the computer or the Internet, the residents themselves could try to assist. At least one community actually implemented this and at times, well after the study was completed, actually requested that our instructors come in for the computer club meetings as a "guest speaker" of sorts. However, getting a club put together took time and effort and relied on a bit of self-governance, and many felt more comfortable with the technical assistance of our study team rather than the assistance of their peers. Offering an ongoing computer class and technical support onsite could motivate residents to continue using the technology, as they will be less likely to be frustrated and give up when they are stuck or have issues with their devices.

In a similar vein, a less frequently cited reason for decreased or discontinued use was accountability:

> Group setting reinforces the lessons ... I won't turn the computer on for another month, but being in the group makes me use the computer 'cause [because it's a set time] (Ms. C., focus group participant).

Some residents noted that the group learning environment and the set schedule of classes motivated them to "stick with it," but without instructors and classmates around to hold them accountable, their technology use would diminish. Again, offering an ongoing computer class or at least an ongoing setting for residents to meet and discuss and troubleshoot the technology together could motivate continued usage.

Other reasons that were mentioned by residents over the course of the study for decreased use include diminishing health or personal matters that needed attending to. Oftentimes, if a resident had an extended stay at the hospital, we would notice that he or she would be less likely to want to "get back into it" and use a computer, as it often required physical and mental exertion beyond what he or she wanted; this perceived exertion was intensified where there was no technical support at the community, as the resident would thus feel like he or she would have to relearn everything independently. Regarding personal matters, there were some residents who simply did not have the time to keep up their current level of usage. As an example, one couple in our study was in the process of selling their old home and moving or selling all of the things that were in the house that they could not store at the CCRC (i.e., their new home). This process took up quite a bit of their time and energy, and thus they felt less inclined to keep up their current level of usage; oftentimes, what free time they had was spent either resting or socializing at the CCRC.

There are thus many reasons for an individual in a CCRC to decrease technology use or to forgo it entirely. Some of these will be out of the control of the CCRC (such as declines in health in the residents). However, continued technology training and the presence of technical support may help in keeping levels of usage up.

5.3   Quality of life outcomes

The term "quality of life" is often used as an umbrella term to describe an individual's overall physical, mental, functional, and social characteristics as well as the individual's satisfaction with these characteristics. The specific dimensions that "quality of life" measures include vary, but it typically involves the intersection between physical, psychological, functional, and social health, and whether or not the individual is content with the current state of his or her health. To illustrate this term, take the hypothetical example of an older adult living in a CCRC who relies on a walker for mobility but is otherwise in excellent physical health. Despite having mobility limitations, this individual may report having a high quality of life if this limitation does not impinge upon recreational and social activities; if the person can still attend meals, go shopping, or visit friends, then the individual may be satisfied with his or her life and thus have a high quality of life. If, however, the walker prevents the individual from being able to carry out daily tasks and attend social activities, the person may report lower levels of quality of life despite the fact that he or she is in excellent physical health. Thus, quality of life is subjective and influenced by a variety of personal factors. One primary focus of technology research has been to evaluate the effect of technology use on measures of quality of life. In this section, we describe findings that show how technology training can improve the quality of life of older adults and, more specifically, the quality of life of older adults living in CCRCs.

5.3.1   Depression and loneliness

One early study that examined the effects of ICT training in retirement communities found that those who received computer training (compared to a control group that did not) trended toward lower levels of depression and loneliness (for more information, see the 1999 and 2002 papers by White and colleagues, which are listed in the Recommended Readings section). Other studies had similar results that suggest that Internet use among older adults was associated with lower levels of depression and loneliness. Presumably, using the Internet gives older adults the capability to stay in touch with friends and family and helps maintain social ties and social support, which in turn helps prevent depression and feelings of loneliness. In theory, using the Internet also gives older adults unprecedented access to treatment and management information that they may use to combat the symptoms of depression and loneliness.

Examining depression and loneliness and how technology use may affect them was a central focus of our study. At the conclusion of our interventions, we wanted to determine whether our results would be similar to those in other studies. For depression, we used survey questions that are a part of commonly used scales that help to determine whether an older adult is experiencing symptoms of depression, such as the following:

- Are you basically satisfied with your life?
- Do you feel pretty worthless the way you are now?
- Do you often feel helpless?
- Do you prefer to stay at home rather than go out and do new things?
- Do you often get bored?

What we found in our study was that CCRC residents who went online several times a week were *less depressed* compared to those who did not go online at all, a finding that is consistent with other studies examining older adults. It would appear that, even in CCRCs, using technologies such as the Internet can have a positive impact with regard to mental well-being.

To determine if learning to use a computer and the Internet was associated with residents feeling less lonely, we examined how frequency of going on the Internet may have a relationship with loneliness, social isolation, and contact with others. In our study, *loneliness* was conceptualized as how often the participants felt lonely, whereas *social isolation* was conceptualized as how often the participants were bothered by not seeing enough of people who were important to them; contact with others was conceptualized as how much the participants felt that the Internet impacted aspects of their social interactions (thus these three measures, although similar, examined different aspects of social life). We found that frequency of going online did not affect social isolation (e.g., Internet use did not decrease how often they were bothered by not seeing close contacts). However, there was a significant impact on loneliness such that the more a participant indicated that he or she went online, the lower were his or her feelings of loneliness. We also found that the more a participant went online, the more likely he or she was to agree that the Internet:

- Made it easier to reach people
- Contributed to the ability to stay in touch with people
- Made it easier to meet new people
- Increased the quantity of communication with others
- Made the participant feel less isolated
- Helped the participant feel more connected to friends and family
- Increased the quality of communication with others

Our results were consistent with previous research that has shown that technology training and interventions designed for older adults can help decrease feelings of loneliness.

5.3.2   Psychological well-being

Although the term "psychological well-being," like the umbrella term "quality of life," can encompass a number of different dimensions, there are six dimensions that are often thought to contribute to an individual's sense of personal happiness and satisfaction (see Ryff (1989), listed in the Recommended Readings section, for further information). These dimensions include the following:

- *Autonomy.* The ability to be self-determinant, independent, and not easily swayed by social pressures.
- *Environmental mastery.* Having control of surrounding situations and an ability to capitalize on opportunities when they arise.
- *Personal growth.* Being open to new experiences and wanting to continually improve oneself.
- *Positive relations to others.* Having "warm and trusting" relationships and an understanding of the "give-and-take" these relationships entail.
- *Purpose in life.* Having a direction and/or goals for living and attaching importance and meaning to both past and present circumstances.
- *Self-acceptance.* Viewing oneself in a positive light and feeling positive about past personal circumstances.

Studies that examined the relationship between Internet use and psychological well-being in older adults found that Internet users, compared to nonusers, tended to score higher on *personal growth* and *purpose in life*. Internet users tended to be more open to new experiences as well as be more likely to have life goals when compared to nonusers. Recent work by Berkowsky (2012, 2014) also examined the relationship between Internet use and the various dimensions of psychological well-being (although it should be noted that these studies did not examine CCRC populations specifically, but instead the general older adult population). Internet users, compared to nonusers, exhibited better psychological well-being, particularly with regard to *personal growth* and *purpose in life* (consistent with earlier studies).

In our study, we did not directly assess the typical six aspects of psychological well-being listed above. However, upon reviewing our field notes and focus group write-ups, we did find evidence that technological interventions and using technologies in CCRCs can increase psychological well-being. The following quote illustrates this point:

> We don't feel like such misplaced people anymore. We know how to Google. We're modern (Ms. W., focus group participant).

Despite being a short quote, it speaks to various dimensions of psychological well-being, such as personal growth (knowing how to Google) and self-acceptance (not feeling misplaced). Statements such as these were frequent when we interviewed participants during and after the trainings, referencing increases in feelings of independence and control thanks to technology (autonomy, environmental mastery), positive attitudes toward learning technology (personal growth), more friendships online and offline (positive relations to others), having more goals and direction as a result of knowing how to use technology (purpose in life), and feeling positive about life in general (self-acceptance).

5.3.3   Spatial and social barriers and connecting with others

During the course of the technology training, we found that moving into a CCRC presents residents with a host of constraints, both real and perceived, that can affect quality of life. These constraints can be both spatial and social in nature. With regard to spatial (or physical) barriers, older adults living in CCRCs may lack the mobility or the transportation that allows them to carry out daily tasks or engage with others— as an example, an older adult who has moved into a CCRC may lack the transportation needed to attend a religious service at the church the resident used to frequent and thus may not visit with old friends. Social barriers, as defined by Winstead et al. (2013), are "the cognitive and social constraints, real or perceived, which may result in reduced social connection and reduced quality of life" (p. 542). These can include cognitive impairment that hinders the development of new friendships in the community or difficulties in developing trust and ease with new residents in the CCRC. In short, moving into a CCRC can create an isolating environment for the resident that promotes feelings of loneliness and unhappiness.

We found that the technology training that was offered allowed residents to increase their technology skills to a point where they were able to overcome these spatial and social barriers. An example of overcoming spatial barriers comes from our study, where one resident used Google Maps Strcct View to look at an old property where she used to live (in seeing the property, she exclaimed, "They cut down my pine trees!" but was overall extremely happy). Another resident used Google to search for websites related to her old church and other areas related to her hometown and remarked, "I feel like I visited home today." In overcoming social barriers, many participants in our study and other communities would remark how email allowed them to stay in better contact with friends and family; as an example, one participant noted how she used email to keep in touch with people from her old church.

5.3.4 Case study—Ms. W.: Transcending spatial and social barriers

One of the more striking examples of technology being used to transcend both spatial and social barriers came from Ms. W., an 87-year-old woman living alone in the assisted living section of the CCRC. She had never been married, had no children, and had no other living family; she had a close friend in whom she liked to confide, but she was no longer able to visit this individual in person. Like other CCRC residents, her entire world was contained within the community—all meals, all activities, all social interactions occurred in that building (or at least what activities she *did* participate in, as other residents remarked that they typically did not see her participate in anything). The portrait of Ms. W. is one that is applicable to many CCRC residents across the country—of being alone and unable to interact with previously valued social contacts.

Despite the isolation Ms. W. may have felt, our interactions with her tended to be quite lively, and we quickly found out that she could be very outgoing and humorous. During one technology training class, the instructor asked the participants about topics they would like to search for using an Internet search engine; when asked what she would like to "look up," Ms. W. quickly responded "A man!" For most, Ms. W. tended to be a source of at least a few giggles.

One day during an office hours session, Ms. W. came in with a mission. She indicated to us that after learning about search engines in class, she wanted to know if she would be able to use something like Google to "look up" people. We informed her that you could use Google to try to search for information on individuals but that there were also some sites, such as www.yellowpages.com, that may be able to provide contact information for someone if she was looking to get in touch with another person. Ms. W. then went on to say that over the course of the class, she was reminded of a dear friend she had grown up with but with whom she had had no contact since high school, and she was wondering if it would be possible to use Google or a site like www.yellowpages.com to try and find this person and reestablish contact with him. We replied that this was possible but that it might be challenging. We sat down with her and began helping her search for her old friend.

We initially began as we did with all office hours sessions, with Ms. W. turning on the computer, logging in, and navigating to the Internet. Once there, we attempted to use Google to find information on her friend but to no avail. We then proceeded to navigate to yellowpages.com to try and find information on him but ran into trouble—because it had been so long since Ms. W. had been in touch with this man, she was unsure as to where he lived. This posed a problem, because a search of this man's name provided numerous search results of men living across the whole country. At this point, Ms. W. indicated that she knew that the man had once lived somewhere in Arizona but that she believed he had moved away from there a long time ago. With nothing else to go on, we reconducted the search on yellowpages.com and narrowed the results to those with addresses in Arizona. Unfortunately, there was no man by that name currently living in Arizona.

In looking at the list of search results, there were a few names that were *close* to that of the man Ms. W. was looking for, but not an exact match. One of the names caught Ms. W.'s eye, or more accurately, the title of one of the names: "Dr." Ms. W. indicated that she knew that the man she was looking for had a son and that he was a physician, and the age of the son would be roughly the same as the "Dr." they found in this search. We quickly conducted a Google search using the name of this physician and found out that this man had a medical practice in Arizona. Ms. W. found the physician's contact information from the main site for the practice and emailed him, asking whether he was who she thought he might be and whether his father was still alive (and whether she could have his contact information if he was). At this point, office hours were coming to a close, and so we had Ms. W. log off of the computer and wished her luck in getting in touch with her long-lost friend.

This case study has a happy ending, as we found out at the next class session that the physician responded to Ms. W. and indicated that he was, in fact, the person she thought he was, and he forwarded the phone number for his father. Ms. W. then proceeded to call her long-lost friend, and they talked for the first time in decades. She was incredibly happy about this interaction to the point of tears. In this instance, Ms. W. was able to successfully use technology to transcend the spatial and social barriers of living in a CCRC and reconnect with an old friend. Ms. W. would later remark in another class session:

> I'm a hot, 87-year-old computer expert. I know how to Google!

5.4   Tech training and understanding as a benefit unto itself

> You can never learn too much—you can always use more (Ms. O., focus group participant).

The above quote was taken from one of our participants during a focus group session conducted after the community had completed our technology training intervention. The quote helps to illustrate the notion that although technology training has the potential to benefit older adult users on a number of quality-of-life outcomes, the process of learning and the knowledge that is gained over the course of training, as well as the experience of participating in a technology class, can be viewed as a benefit unto itself. Simply put, the act of learning something new can provide a sense of accomplishment—even if the participant has no intention of using the technology after the class is complete.

> I may be old, but I feel like I've accomplished something...my whole family has computers, I feel like I've accomplished something (Ms. P., focus group participant).
>
> I'm 88 years old, I have 11 grandchildren, they talked about things I didn't know what it was...now I can understand what they are talking about. It made me feel good (Ms. M., focus group participant).

Although having the knowledge of how to successfully use many different technologies was an oft-cited benefit among the participants of our study, just *having* knowledge at all about the technologies (regardless of being able to successfully apply that knowledge) was sometimes enough for participants to have an overwhelming sense of accomplishment and satisfaction. Many participants were happy with learning the terminology of computer and Internet use, as this helped them with being able to keep up in discussions with friends and family.

> I learned a lot of terminology. We learned the language (Ms. S., focus group participant).
>
> I took this course because I read the techno column in the paper and [now] understand what they were talking about (Ms. McC., focus group participant).

This benefit was most apparent with regard to social networking. On numerous occasions we would have participants indicate to us that they would see a news broadcast or commercial that requested the viewer to "like us on Facebook" or "follow us on Twitter," and the participants would have no idea what "like" or "follow" meant in this context. After the class sessions, however, they would have an understanding of this terminology and thus would know exactly what these broadcasts and commercials were referring to. The participants experienced a level of satisfaction with being able to understand what was being discussed around them.

5.5   Conclusion

There is a wide variety of benefits associated with conducting a technology training course in a CCRC, including (but not limited to) promoting more positive attitudes toward technology, increasing self-efficacy, promoting increased technology use, increasing quality of life, increasing technology knowledge, and giving residents a sense of accomplishment. All things considered, older adults in CCRCs may greatly benefit from a technology training course that is provided to them in the CCRC setting. However, these benefits may be short term without continued training and support, and thus CCRCs should be prepared to offer ongoing programs or individual assistance to ensure that these benefits remain constant among residents.

Recommended readings

Berkowsky, R. W., Cotten, S. R., Yost, E. A., and Winstead, V. P. 2013. Attitudes towards and limitations to ICT use in assisted and independent living communities: Findings from a specially-designed technological intervention. *Educational Gerontology, 39,* 797–811.

Cody, M. J., Dunn, D., Hoppin, S., and Wendt, P. 1999. Silver surfers: Training and evaluating Internet use among older adult learners. *Communication Education, 48,* 269–286.

Heo, J., Chun, S., Lee, S., Lee, K. H., and Kim, J. 2015. Internet use and well-being in older adults. *Cyberpsychology, Behavior, and Social Networking, 18*(5), 268–272. doi:10.1089/cyber.2014.0549.

Ryff, C. D. 1989. Happiness is everything, or is it? Explorations on the meaning of psychological well-being. *Journal of Personality and Social Psychology, 57*(6), 1069–1081.

Wagner, N., Hassanein, K., and Head, M. 2010. Computer use by older adults: A multi-disciplinary review. *Computers in Human Behavior, 26,* 870–882.

White, H., McConnell, E., Clipp, E., Branch, L. G., Sloane, R., and Pieper, C. 2002. A randomized controlled trial of the psychosocial impact of providing Internet training and access to older adults. *Aging & Mental Health, 6*(3), 213–221.

White, H., McConnell, E., Clipp, E., Bynum, L., Teague, C., Navas, L., Craven, S., and Halbrecht, H. 1999. Surfing the net in later life: A review of the literature and pilot study of computer use and quality of life. *Journal of Applied Gerontology, 18,* 358–378.

Winstead, V., Anderson, W. A., Yost, E. A., Cotten, S. R., Warr, A., and Berkowsky, R. W. 2013. You can teach an old dog new tricks: A qualitative analysis of how residents of senior living communities may use the Web to overcome spatial and social barriers. *Journal of Applied Gerontology, 32,* 540–560.

chapter six

Recruiting and retaining older adults in technology training programs

Older adults who have never used technology may be difficult to recruit and retain for a technology training program. At their stage of life, they may not see the value in learning to use a computer, the Internet, or any other type of technology. Learning to use such things as the Internet can seem more like work than enjoyment. They have come to a point in their lives where they believe that statements such as "At my age if I don't want to do it, I am NOT going to do it," are true for them. For older adults, learning to use technology might not be worth the hassle of commitment to training sessions and putting forth the effort to learn something new. Because older adults have unique learning challenges, they must be convinced that the training program will be doable and that they can successfully learn without feeling incompetent, unable, or embarrassed about their difficulties with the technology or their initial lack of skill. This chapter addresses issues with both recruitment and retention of older adults in CCRCs for technology training programs. Information garnered from our 5-year longitudinal study has informed best practices in recruitment as well as retention for this unique population. Information can also be generalized to a broader group of older adults in technology training programs or to researchers organizing studies in CCRCs.

6.1 Recruitment

Recruiting older adults to participate in a technology training program can be a challenge in and of itself. Recruiting older adults who live in some form of CCRC can be an even greater challenge because recruitment begins not with the residents themselves but with the community's administration. Although each community will have a different organizational structure, most of the corporate communities follow a model similar to the one shown in Figure 6.1. Administrators must perceive the training program to be useful for residents, not a distraction for the nonparticipants, and as something that does not interfere with or impede other

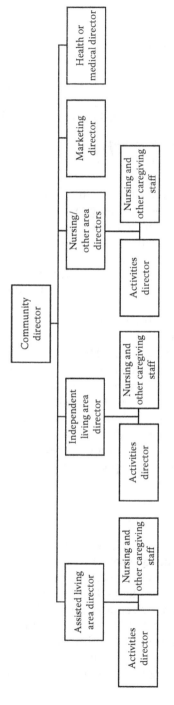

Figure 6.1 Basic organizational structure of administration in a CCRC.

activities provided by the community. They must also view it as beneficial in terms of promoting their community socially to residents who are part of the community and also to prospective new members of the community or others in their corporate system. For example, in a community that participated in our technology training, an administrator attended a couple of the sessions and took photographs to use in promotional literature as a way of marketing the community to potential residents. The photographs were used to show potential community members how residents had opportunities for personal and social growth through activities such as our computer training classes. She also used one of the photographs to display in the front lobby for family members and visitors to see as they entered the assisted living community.

Getting in contact with administrators regarding a new technology training program can provide an unforeseen and unique hurdle, as it is sometimes difficult to get administrators to take the time to return phone calls to set up an initial meeting. Phone calls regarding new activities are usually not effective as a way to connect with administrators as they are not recognized as a priority. Activity directors often prove to be the best initial contact through which to reach administrators. Although their position is not considered to be administrative, activity directors are more accessible and have a greater vested interest than do administrators in providing another activity choice for their residents—simply put, activity directors are more likely to listen compared to the other professionals working at the community.

One of the main jobs of an activity director is to create monthly activity calendars and encourage residents to participate in the activities. One way to do this is to have consistent and innovative activities. Many of these monthly activity calendars are planned and approved months in advance so that residents and families can set schedules. The main purpose of these activities is to promote residents' well-being. Successful activities are seen as ones that are not cost prohibitive, have a high turnout rate, and can be safely implemented in the CCRC. Taking this into account, it was especially helpful to meet face-to-face with the activity directors to show them the benefits to their residents of a technology training program. The recognition that they did not have to contribute to the training program, except to help us recruit, and the fact that the training met the criteria cited, made the training program especially attractive to activity directors.

In short, activity directors can be effective at providing the initial contact with community administrators and thus can be used to set up the first meeting with them. Activity directors can "prime the pump" with administrators by signifying their own approval and showing their willingness to be the liaison with the technology training team. They are invaluable for assisting in the approval and permission process from the administration or to begin the process of getting approval from the larger corporation, if applicable. They are also much more in touch with individual residents; thus, they are useful later on in the recruitment of participants. Often, they will identify residents whom they believe will benefit the most from the training and, conversely, residents for whom training would be stressful and ineffective because of cognitive or physical barriers. As stated in Chapter 4, activity directors are a vital component to a successful technology training program, even in the early stages of recruitment, before any resident even looks at a computer screen.

6.1.1   Recruitment sessions

Recruitment to a technology class can be daunting. Selling many older adults on the benefit and use of technology is rarely done in one meeting. Recruitment can be done in a variety of ways and should employ multiple types of strategies to attract interest in technology training. This section discusses the pros and cons of differing types of recruitment sessions.

In general, to maximize recruitment efforts, several levels of recruitment are important for reaching as many residents as possible. Formal recruitment occurs when there is a scheduled information session that is focused primarily on introducing residents to the proposed training; this can involve having a meeting with residents where the technology classes are the focus of the discussion or can involve "piggybacking" onto an already planned or ongoing activity or presentation. Another option we describe is recruitment tied to family or resident council meetings. Lastly, we discuss informal recruitment or recruitment that is unscheduled, such as dropping by a common area or the dining area to just sit and chat with residents either one-on-one or in small groups.

6.1.1.1   Formal recruitment sessions

Formal recruitment sessions are economical and efficient methods of recruiting in CCRCs. During formal recruitment sessions, maintaining an open dialogue, rather than asking residents to commit to the training, allows residents a pressure-free atmosphere. Residents who might possibly have an interest in the training were asked to sign a sheet that was passed from resident to resident. This was more effective than the residents coming forward to give their contact information after an explanation of the project. Often, residents who initially had no interest provide their contact information because other residents with whom they are friends had signed the sheet; they did not want to feel left out.

We found that it was effective to combine some sort of real activity with the information session, such as providing a musical presentation

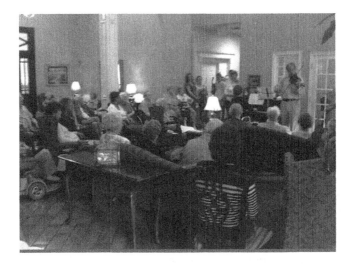

Figure 6.2 Recruitment session with a special music presentation.

with an informational talk about training; such an activity ensured that a greater number of residents would attend compared to advertising an information session. For example, we worked with one activity director to advertise a pianist and violinist as an afternoon activity, combined with short informational presentations about the computer training in between musical numbers. We had a large group of residents attend, and many signed up for more information that day. On another occasion, we attended a musical activity planned by the CCRC for which we provided refreshments (see Figure 6.2). Because the activity was already planned, our informational session was simply an addition to the program; we often referred to this type of recruitment strategy as "piggybacking." This had a similar outcome and provided us with a list of residents who gave us their permission to contact them with more details about the training program.

Although formal, these sessions were mainly a way for residents to get to know study staff and see a little about what the project would entail. The forming of relationships at this step is vital to recruiting the greatest number of participants. The formal recruitment also allowed many residents to ask questions or express concerns that others might not be willing to ask. Several members of the research team were available after these sessions to spend time talking one-on-one with residents following the presentation, which also helped to establish rapport with potential participants.

A major concern expressed by the residents with regard to our training program was making a commitment for 8 weeks of technology training.

Despite many of the residents not having prior computer or Internet experience, many recognized the importance in continuity of class attendance to successfully learn and practice how to work with these new devices, applications, and concepts. Reasons such as doctor's appointments, physical therapy sessions, or regular visitation times with family members were cited as obstacles to participation as the residents were fearful that, should they miss too many classes, they would fall behind without hope of being able to catch up or, potentially worse, being dropped from the class entirely. They needed to be assured of the flexibility of the program; for example, for our study, they could miss up to four sessions during the 8 weeks and still participate in the study. After four absences, they could not participate in future surveys, but they could remain in the class as a participant. If there were concerns about absences and falling behind the rest of the class, they were reminded that we offered an office hours session each week where they would be able to meet with instructors and catch up on any new information or practice what they had already learned.

This latter accommodation was particularly important. In fact, for any training conducted in CCRCs, we advise having optional office hours where participants can drop in to ask questions or catch up on things that they missed or did not fully grasp during training sessions. This is also an additional opportunity for participants to bond with the trainers and with other residents who are participating in the training program.

Even though Chapter 4 discussed considerations and accommodations that can be made to develop a successful technology training program for older adults in CCRCs (taking into account the specific needs of older learners), these accommodations are wasted if residents decide not to participate. In our training program, some expressed concerns about having no prior experience with technology. It may be important, if you have residents with little technology experience, to describe the training program as "starting with the basics" to reassure possible participants that prior knowledge about or exposure to technology is not necessary. We have found this useful in our training activities. Some residents may also express concern about perceived physical or cognitive limitations that might hold the rest of the class back. It is important to handle these concerns in a sensitive manner, as was done by our team members, with assurance given that they would have opportunities for one-on-one help both in class and in between training sessions. We also found it important to reassure participants that they could drop out of the training program at any point with no repercussions. For the most skeptical, we offered the option of attending a class without signing up first to just try it out. We found that if they came the first time, it was very likely they would sign up and stay in the class for the duration.

6.1.1.2   Using family council or other community meetings

Having a separate, formal recruitment session is just one way to encourage participation and recruit participants. Using residents' families and social networks is also useful. Family council meetings occur at most CCRCs four times a year. They serve the purpose of providing updated information about the CCRC, such as new staff, schedule changes, or fee increases, and they are used to address the concerns of family members. Although it may be difficult to plan around these meetings, they can be very rewarding for recruitment sessions. These meetings provide unique opportunities for residents' families to encourage their loved ones to participate. They can remind them of the new possibilities for communication that using information and communication technologies (ICTs) can offer. Residents often must be convinced that it will be enjoyable and useful. They often want to talk it over with a child or other family member to see what they think about the resident's participation. Having a family member's endorsement and encouragement is one of the most effective ways to get residents to want to participate in the training.

Family council meetings, or any meetings in which family members of residents participate, provide an opportunity to talk with both residents and family members about the training. We found it helpful to have residents from other communities who have participated in training speak briefly about their own experience with computer, Internet, or other technology use at the council meetings and the training classes that we offered. This gave both residents and their families the opportunity to hear a resident from another CCRC talk about the benefits of using technology. After the informational sessions, it is useful to have the residents from other communities who participated in the training program be available to sit with individual residents and/or their family members and answer questions and perhaps even allay fears or concerns they may have about the training process. Many older adults have difficulty visualizing themselves as computer users at their stage of life, so having someone who is their peer and a successful computer user can be advantageous. In this, they not only see how technology training has been beneficial for their peers, but also can have encouragement from their families and see what new avenues of communication and support they receive from them.

6.1.1.3   Informal recruitment sessions

It is important to provide materials that show the benefit of the training to the CCRC and to the individual residents. We found that providing hard copies of information, such as a pamphlet or flyer that describes the program in detail, were effective because residents have something to read, take home with them, show to their relatives, and think about after we spoke to them. Many residents did not want to make an immediate decision about participating; having something that gave an overview of the study along with contact information for study personnel was helpful.

As a follow-up in several communities, we dropped by during a mealtime or an activity and sat with individual residents to chat about the training and the benefits to them individually. We found that establishing these relationships early was effective in both recruiting and retaining residents. This also provided us the opportunity to show our own enthusiasm in providing the training to them. It was important that they viewed us as enthusiastic, positive, and supportive of their ability to be successful in learning how to use technology.

Materials that are provided for recruitment purposes should be specifically geared toward older adults and what is known about their attitudes toward technology. Materials should include pictorial representations of how *they* can use the computer to stay in touch—for example, a picture of an older adult talking to a grandchild on Skype or FaceTime or "walking" down his or her former street on Google Street View. During the recruitment session, it is helpful to have personally relevant examples of the benefits of computer training, such as setting up a computer with a slideshow of pictures. Being able to see this can be effective in providing the older adults with a tangible representation of the benefits to them of being a technology user. Residents who signed up for our training program were intrigued with the idea of having a way of receiving pictures of family members and especially grandchildren. For an example of recruitment material, see Figure 6.3.

Older adults may believe that technology has no relevance for their lives or that they are too old to take on the challenge of learning something new. The description of the training process must be thorough and clearly presented in both the oral presentation and in the recruitment materials if such beliefs are to be countered.

6.1.2   Special considerations for recruiting in research settings

In their discussion on recruiting older adults for research, McNeely and Clements (1994) note that participation in research is highest for younger populations and declines as people age. Recruitment and retention for research can be especially difficult for older adults in CCRCs. One strategy is to avoid the word "research" because of the association of the word with abuses in the past before regulations were put into place to protect human subjects who participated in research. We tried to minimize presenting the training as a research project during recruitment while emphasizing the training as a positive activity that was beneficial to their

Timothy Gill on Violin
Join us for a musical event and presentation
May 4th @2:00 in the living room!

Grantswood University
(fictitious name to preserve anonymity of sites) presents a
musical event of light classics featuring Tim Gill on
Violin and Vicki Gill on piano.

Immediately following, there will be a short
presentation on a computer training opportunity for
residents!

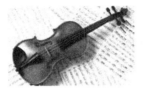

Figure 6.3 Example of a recruitment flyer linked with an entertainment session.

well-being. Although we avoided the word "research" in our general recruitment sessions and materials, the overall goals and purpose of the project were clearly stated in the consent documents to ensure that the residents understood that it was a research project and they were agreeing to participate.

For researchers, informed consent is something needed in almost all research involving human subjects, particularly if it is funded by a government agency or foundation. If the training is not part of a research project, informed consent documents may not be needed. An informed consent document gives research participants all necessary information for the study they are about to enter. It informs them of information that is asked of them as participants and provides details of any possible risks to participating in the research.

One issue researchers might encounter is the ability to make sure that the document is understood by the participant. There can be underlying cognitive or other issues that result in the participant not being able to completely understand the full document. Though this type of research is likely to cause no harm, ICTs can make this population more susceptible to predation than others. When providing participants with the informed consent document, it is often good to go over it section-by-section and offer time after each section for questions and explanations. Reading the document to the individual is not enough. Time and care must be taken to ensure he or she understands each section. Often, returning another day after going over the document in-depth is a good idea. Although participants may choose not to do another review of the materials on a later day, it made them feel more comfortable to have this option.

One unique issue, specific to ICT training programs, is the issue of online security. As older adults learn to use ICTs, it is very important to remember to teach them basic safety measures for online information as well. Scams are often targeted at this age group, and it is the duty of the researchers to inform the participants to the best of their ability. All of this should be included in the informed consent document, and the participants should be made aware of the possibilities (and the training should include information about how to minimize risks).

6.1.3   Recruiting at different care levels of the CCRC

At their basic structural organization, CCRCs are composed of levels of care for independent living (IL), assisted living (AL), special care assisted living for residents with dementia, and skilled nursing. The various levels are housed on the same campus, but the level of care provided in each differs in need, abilities, and approaches. As CCRCs entail multiple levels of care, there may be different approaches in recruitment for different levels. Older adults in independent living tend to be healthier and somewhat younger. Although they are usually no longer working, they might be involved in various activities such as volunteer work, church- or religious-based activities, traveling, or family involvement. Although they may not have the same types of activities they had in the past, the independent living residents who are more likely to consent to participate are also involved in other types of activities. The myth that older adults have a lot of spare time did not prove to be true for our technology study. For example, one of our female independent living participants made time for the training, but surveys that were a part of the research were difficult to schedule because she volunteered for her church and helped her daughter by taking her grandchildren to and from school each day.

Assisted living residents tend to be older and frailer than their independent living counterparts. Their consent to participate may be hindered by their health status. Daily life may require the majority of their energy, and performing activities of daily living may be overwhelming and all that can be achieved. Medical appointments often consume a great deal of time. It is difficult to direct energy to learning something new when struggling to get through the day physically. Therefore, during recruitment, reminding these individuals of the ability to miss a class or two is important. It takes a great burden off of them in thinking that they are not required to be there every class and that they can make up any missed topic during office hours.

Table 6.1 Summary of recruitment recommendations

Recruitment recommendations
• Recruit through multiple avenues—formal and informal sessions, and larger family events
• Emphasize the flexibility and learner-friendly design of the program
• Develop positive relationships with activity directors in CCRCs
• Highlight senior-centric benefits of technology use
• Develop recruitment strategies that cater to specific needs of residents, based on the level of care

Table 6.1 summarizes the recommendations given above.

Although it may be possible to conduct a variety of types of technology trainings in specialty care assisted living facilities and skilled nursing sections of CCRCs, we do not focus on these sections as the physical and mental constraints of residents are generally vastly different from those in the AL and IL sections. Our experiences have been in working with AL and IL residents. In addition, we have seen few published studies detailing research-focused technology interventions in specialty care assisted living and nursing sections of CCRCs.

6.2   Retention

Once the initial hurdles of recruitment have been overcome, keeping older adults in technology classes can be difficult. Retaining them in the training is important on two fronts: it is important that they attend all classes, or at least most training sessions to (1) benefit from learning the new technology and (2) obtain accurate and meaningful study outcomes (i.e., if the technology training is a component of a research study). The remainder of this chapter addresses key findings in relation to aspects of participant retention. We address retention in terms of needs, rapport, class time, and office hours. It is best to be in tune with the older adults' needs (physical, emotional, social, and cognitive) throughout the training. Having an understanding of these areas for each participant is fundamental to maintaining the relationship throughout the training duration. Building rapport with residents will help researchers understand the unique needs of each resident for the learning process. Further, organizing the training to work well as a learning environment for multiple types of learners is crucial. To ensure this, having time both in class and outside of class, using multiple examples for each topic area, being consistent and clear with directions, and having time for questions are important. Each of these aspects are evaluated below.

6.2.1   Needs

Chapter 4 discussed *general* accommodations technology trainers can make in preparing a class for CCRC residents. But although researchers may have some awareness of any physical needs a participant enters the study with, *individual abilities can change over the course of a few weeks or months.* Constant monitoring is needed. Can the participant hear the instructor? Can the participant see the text on the screen? Is the participant having dexterity issues? Is there a time of day that seems to be better for the participant? Although researchers cannot adapt to every need, knowing how each of the physical needs will impact the likelihood of the participant continuing is key. As soon as issues are noted, steps to correct them are necessary. Perhaps, Mrs. C. recently got injections for macular degeneration. Her vision will be compromised a bit. However, text size and brightness of the screen can be adjusted. There are additional programs that can be installed to help her continue to use the computer. If Mr. M.'s hearing aid is not working well enough, move him to the front of the room, facing the instructor. Perhaps, when the weather changes, Mrs. B.'s arthritis causes more dexterity problems; offer her options to make typing or using the mouse easier. Even small physical changes can throw participants off and cause them to withdraw from the training out of fear of looking or feeling incompetent.

Emotional needs are more difficult to assess. However, attention and planning are essential to successfully retaining participants. With ICTs, there is a danger of the skills being considered complex and difficult to learn, either for the first time or for newer or different technology. The researchers should make clear that frustration is normal but can be overcome. The feelings of self-doubt can negatively impact study findings or play into a self-fulfilling prophecy if participants feel they will be unable to learn or retain what they have learned. Emotional needs that show themselves during the training can be dealt with in part by knowing the participants and their stories and through reassurance from study leaders to participants. The time that our research team spent pretraining really helped here. Surveys that were administered pretraining offered one-on-one time between research team members and residents, which helped to build rapport. Thirty-minute surveys often turned into 60–90 minutes of time spent with a resident. This allowed our team to get to know the person's history, why they had moved into the CCRC, and their daily struggles. In follow-up surveys, residents even requested that a particular team member administer the survey because of relationships that were forged.

Social needs are one of the more interesting complications of community living. Groups are a natural part of human life; humans form and reform them often. CCRCs are just another setting in which this occurs.

When forming seating charts or helping make sure participants are comfortable, take into account the social networks present in their community and in their group (if the training is being done as part of a study). Placing individuals who do not get along at the same table, or in close proximity, might have adverse outcomes on retention of participants. Knowing the participants and making the training participant-centered will help overcome these issues should they arise. On the positive side, we found that new friendships and groups formed because of participants' time together over the 8 weeks that our trainings lasted.

Cognitive barriers should be assessed prior to the initial training. However, as time progresses, illness occurs, medications change, and other stressors can result in cognitive issues. Although significant cognitive changes typically do not happen overnight, if the project is ongoing, trainers may see some cognitive change. It might be so mild it is difficult to spot at first. Though it is difficult to know when the cognitive decline has so affected the person that it is no longer possible for him or her to continue in the training program, small changes can build upon one another. As we recognized a particular struggle a resident might have, we tried to be proactive in offering assistance. For example, we knew Ms. S. had trouble hearing and so one helper stayed close by to "parrot" instructions that were being given. Ms. R. had trouble remembering her password for her email account, so we wrote it in a prominent place in her manual.

Adding extra precautions at the beginning of the project, such as using a basic cognitive screener (Mini Mental Status Examination [MMSE] is one example), can mitigate some larger problems later. A basic cognitive screener assesses various components of cognitive decline that might interfere with the ability to retain new information. For research, an MMSE might also be useful after training or at later points in time to quantify any changes researchers are seeing in the participant. Knowing participants and maintaining a relationship with them throughout the training program is key in addressing issues of retention in the project.

6.2.2   Building rapport

All of the needs discussed above can be addressed through the relationship the training team builds with the participant. Knowing the participant, their background, their history, and so on will allow for a relationship to develop and for trust to be built. We found it to be helpful to stop, sit, and listen. This was accomplished by arriving early at the CCRC so that we would have the opportunity to spend time with individual residents outside of the training session. Often, we stayed after the session and visited with individuals or groups of residents. *Learning their names and calling them by their names is extremely important.* If they believe that they are nothing more than a research subject or study participant, they will be less engaged and at a higher risk for dropping out. Being willing to ask questions about their day or week and then being willing to listen helped residents to feel connected to us. This relationship and trust are crucial in retaining participants. In our study, participants would occasionally tell us that they "really didn't feel like participating today" but that they came regardless because they told us they would.

In CCRCs, there are multiple levels of care. Some of the residents have few to no physical or cognitive issues and require no additional support, whereas others have significant physical or cognitive needs and require much more support. Treating all of the participants with respect, and not infantilizing them as you explain the technology, is important. When teaching, speak to the participants as adults and avoid "elderspeak"—a change in communication patterns when speaking to older adults that tends to cause communication patterns to be more simplistic, overly endearing, and repetitive. This type of communication can be patronizing and reinforces stereotypes of aging, thus alienating participants from trainers. Avoiding this is key in building rapport.

Another way to develop rapport is treating participants as equals in the learning process. To help with this, make sure participants complete the tasks by themselves. It will seem easier to help them move the mouse or make one small change for them, but that does not help the participants learn and it does not help them build the confidence needed to complete the task. Ensuring that they learn how to navigate each task independently means they have to learn how to troubleshoot and be confident in their abilities. This often means talking them through tasks, such as opening and closing programs multiple times, in a calm and patient manner. Building rapport with participants is paramount to the success of the intervention.

6.2.3   Class time

Once participants are in class, everything should be done to meet their physical, emotional, social, and cognitive needs and, when possible, meet their needs without them having to ask. Class time should be structured yet flexible, fun, productive, informative, and encouraging, and should offer a glimpse as to why what they are learning is useful or important to them. This will increase the likelihood that participants will want to continue coming back to class and participating in the study or training program.

Making learning fun is important for any learning activity at any age. When learning a new technology through a formal classroom setting, the activities must be fun. Even if the material is challenging to learn, activities can be designed around participants' likes and dislikes. When learning how to send attachments, specific files (e.g., fun pictures) were used to make the class enjoyable. Participants uploaded and attached one of two pictures and sent it to one or more of their classmates, so everyone saw both pictures before the class was over. When learning how to search YouTube, suggestions from participants were taken to learn what they would like to see in terms of videos.

Class time can be made fun by making sure there is a structure, but allowing the class to diverge from a topic when needed. One rather poignant experience for our study came from a woman receiving an email from her granddaughter at the beginning of class. Although that class time was meant to be used for another topic, the email from this granddaughter included a picture of the sonogram of what would be the participant's first great-grandchild. Instead of pushing on with the lecture planned for the day, we allowed the participant to share the picture with the class by forwarding it to her classmates. This made the class more enjoyable to her and reinforced how to forward messages with attachments. The ability to make class time fun ties back into knowing your participants.

Showing participants the role ICTs can have in their lives is particularly important for this age group and for participants in this type of training (whether in a research setting or not). On more than one occasion, researchers in our study heard that potential participants did not need this type of learning or these types of devices. Prior to participation, many people did not feel that this was really something that would prove useful to them. This was often one of the larger battles fought in this type of program. However, upon completion of the training program, there was an overwhelming feeling of accomplishment and pride in completing and knowing how to use the new technology. Many respondents further reported that they felt connected to the world in ways they had not previously felt connected. The ICT knowledge allowed them to overcome barriers that their age, health status, and living arrangements presented them with. Using ICTs could allow them to virtually walk down their childhood streets, visit museums in other countries, speak to relatives who lived far away, connect with individuals from their past, and keep up with family and friends in new ways. These results are discussed in detail in Chapter 5, but the key point to reiterate here is that these benefits will increase retention. Find ways to show participants early on that this type of knowledge and these skills will benefit them. This also speaks to the skills you are trying to impart. The skills younger generations might need to know for basic computer literacy are different from the skills older adults will need for basic computer literacy. Making sure that the skills are clearly defined and suited for the specific target demographic is essential in retaining participants.

Making classroom directions clear and repeating them frequently plays into retention in technology training programs. Specifically for older adults, directions must be repeated and given in a loud and clear voice. Make sure the instructor has an easy-to-understand voice and enunciates well. The noise from multiple computers and a classroom full of people makes it difficult for most people to hear. For older adults who might already have hearing issues and not be familiar with key terms, having someone who is loud and clear is important. It will reduce frustration for the participants and hopefully keep the class time productive for the participants.

Furthermore, giving directions in the same manner for each skill is vital. As participants learn from repeated attempts at an activity, directions should be given in the same steps, using the same key terms each time. We found that the slightest change, from a different instructor giving directions, or the same instructor giving options for steps, often confused participants. Once an instructor has been chosen, it is often best to stay with one instructor for continuity and familiarity. Directions are more likely to be given in the same manner each time, and the participants can find comfort in seeing the same face each time. Frequent, clear directions reduce frustrations and keep participants engaged in class material, thus reducing dropout from the training program or study.

In learning how to manage new technologies, one-on-one attention can be vital in helping individuals master the skills necessary to use the class time well. In our study, each class session had two to four floating assistants (usually graduate students) to make sure all participants were where they needed to be and were not falling behind. This type of individual attention can be beneficial in that no one will get so far behind that they will not be able to catch up. Floaters also provide the personal attention many participants seek in this type of learning environment. Floaters can help personalize each lesson for the participant and keep the participant's interest peaked for each session. However, it is important to maintain the autonomy of the participants. The floaters should not do the skills for the participants. No matter how far behind or how difficult the task, the participant should complete the task on his or her own. This builds self-efficacy in the participant and allows him or her to be active learners.

Lastly, in terms of class time, instructors and other training personnel should be encouraging at all times. They should use positive language and not shy away or simply do a task for someone who is struggling. Participants should feel encouraged throughout their time in class. Some of the material will be difficult, but constant encouragement and positive language will go far for the learner. This can often be difficult, especially if one person falls behind. The natural stance is to want to get the individual caught up by doing a task for him or her. Some participants might even request that tasks be done for them. However, encouraging the participants to do it for themselves is key in retaining them as participants. If they feel that tasks get too difficult or they are asking for too much help, they will likely not return to class. (It is also worthwhile to remind them of the availability of office hours for refresher training if they seem frustrated or uncertain.)

The key things to remember for class time include the following: participants are happiest and most likely to continue when class time is flexible and fun, and the reason they are learning a concept is clear; class time is informative and productive; and participants are constantly encouraged. Having a good understanding of your participants and building rapport with them will help ensure that class time is beneficial for both participants and trainers.

6.2.4 Office hours

Another method for personalizing technology training and reinforcing learned tasks is through holding office hours. Office hours are simply times that researchers or other trainers are available for participants to practice new skills or explore other topics not covered in class. For our office hours, participants often wanted to learn more in-depth functions of websites, reinforce what they had learned, or simply be able to explore while having someone there for support. Having office hours each week during training and then for a few weeks post-training is key for participants being able to retain the knowledge, move ahead, and personalize the skills they wish to gain out of the training program.

Because office hours are a time for one-on-one training, many participants took advantage of this time. If they had missed a class or two and were feeling behind, this was a time they could come and catch up on what they had missed and perhaps get ahead or reinforce prior weeks' class topics. This personalized tailoring helps meet needs, allows individuals to explore topics of personal interest, and helps show them that the technology can be beneficial for their lives. Although the majority of people who showed up to office hours during our training sessions wanted to work directly on the computers, we also had some participants come to office hours merely to watch others use the computers and to hear the types of questions they were asking. In this way, they were learning vicariously by watching their classmates learn new things and/or practice things they had already learned in the training sessions.

Table 6.2 summarizes our recommendations for retention.

Table 6.2 Summary of retention recommendations

Retention recommendations
• Address as many physical needs of participants as possible
• Attempt to address emotional needs and frustrations as soon as they arise
• Build rapport with the participants
• Get feedback from participants in class to make learning applicable and fun
• Set aside time outside of class to address individual questions, concerns, and to allow for additional supervised practice
• Provide opportunities for participants to catch up on training if they miss a training session

6.3   The role of the activity director in recruitment and retention

The activity director can be a crucial component of recruitment and retention. However, not all activity directors are created equal. We found that the activity director in each community played a role to varying degrees in the daily life of the residents. In addition, we found that there is a high turnover rate among activity directors (at least the ones in the 19 communities that we were involved with during the course of our multiyear project). This is difficult for residents and can make it especially difficult in recruitment and retention. Having an activity director who will work with you to optimize the time, space, and resident involvement is crucial. We worked with several activity directors who had extensive knowledge about the lives, personalities, and habits of their residents, more so than other staff or administrators. When the activity director has a positive relationship with the residents, the residents are more likely to participate in activities that are provided or endorsed by the activity director. Get the activity director involved in recruitment and in the implementation of the training sessions. Two polar extremes of activity directors that demonstrate their efficacy can be found in the following examples.

At one CCRC, the activity director was labeled by research staff as the "queen of activity directors." The close relationship she shared with her residents was evident from the first time we met her. She lovingly referred to the residents as "her guys." They saw her advocating for them with the administration when there were circumstances with which they were unhappy. In turn, the residents described her as their friend and represented their feelings toward their community at large. As one resident described daily life,

> (She) has a whole evening prepared...lined up for
> us. She's wonderful... She cares for us and she sees

> that you're looked after. This place is dead when she's out (Ms. M., 85-year-old AL participant).

Another resident expressed a similar sentiment:

> Well, it's been...we've had a wonderful director, Candace. Candace has been our director and I have just loved her. She is the most talented little lady you ever saw... Candace has planned nice things for us from time to time, something that you enjoy and she has faced each day. It's just that she, she's just a key effect... when she's not here, everything is just sort of, sort of silent (Ms. G., 95-year-old AL participant).

At a different community, the activity director took a more hands-off approach. She had been rotated into the position recently. She was working part time as the activity director and part time in a job outside the CCRC. She was stretched for time and put together childish and mundane activities for the residents. Many residents we spoke with reported that they tried to attend a few of her activities but felt like they were being talked down to when they engaged with her. Many reported not knowing her. Even by the end of the 8 weeks of our training program, most residents at the CCRC had spent more time engaging with our staff than with their own activity director.

Our point in making these distinctions is that activity directors will vary in their engagement with residents and in how effective they may be in helping you recruit for your training program. Do not assume that all activity directors will be as engaged and helpful as Candace, whom we described above. However, when you have one as engaged as Candace, it is a great asset to any program you may be trying to conduct in a CCRC.

6.4 Role of incentives in recruitment and retention for research projects

Researchers have investigated the importance and necessity of incentives for keeping individuals engaged in research projects, and guidelines have emerged. The type and size of incentive should be carefully considered. Monetary incentives are always popular, but the way in which they are provided can be instrumental in their being viewed as beneficial or not. Although many participants in our study/training program reported not wanting or needing the incentives to keep them engaged, many appreciated them. Gift cards are popular with younger groups and are typically easy to use, track, and distribute. However, for older adults, there seems to be much hesitation behind the use of gift cards. There is often confusion about how to use them, when to use them, and where to use them. Therefore, the gift cards provided as incentives were often viewed as difficult to use or not worth it. Cash incentives or checks are recommended in that these methods are easier for participants to use and cause less frustration and confusion for many older adults. Having a good sense of your potential participants will help you decide if you need to provide incentives; and, if provided, what the most appropriate types of incentives are. Activity directors can also be helping in determining appropriate incentives for training programs.

Financial incentives may be useful and affect participation, but participants also have many internal incentives for completing these programs. Although each participant will have different internal motivations, we often reminded participants of the new skills they were gaining, how they could easily find information online they might need, and how great it was to surprise their families with their new methods of communication. Participants reported feeling more connected to the world after learning many of these skills, something a financial incentive cannot buy.

6.5 Conclusion

The organizational complexity and unique populations of CCRCs create challenges that require special attention for potential researchers and trainers. To achieve the goals of the program, great care should be taken during recruitment. Hosting formal and informal recruitment sessions, planning ahead, and getting support from the activity director is crucial for a successful recruitment. To retain participants, special needs should be addressed early and evaluated often. Maintaining a strong relationship not only with participants but also with management and community leaders, such as activity directors, is necessary for a successful training program or study.

Recommended readings

Davies, S. L., Goodman, C., Manthorpe, J., Smith, A., Carrick, N., and Iliffe, S. 2014. Enabling research in care homes: An evaluation of a national network of research ready care homes. *BMC Medical Research Methodology*, 14, 47. doi: 10.1186/1471-2288-14-47.

McHenry, J. C., Insel, K. C., Einstein, G. O., Vidrine, A. N., Koerner, K. M., and Morrow, D. G. 2015. Recruitment of older adults: Success may be in the details. *The Gerontologist*, 55(5), 845–853.

McNeely, E. A. and Clements, S. D. 1994. Recruitment and retention of the older adults into research studies. *Journal of Neuroscience Nursing*, 26, 57–61.

Reich, W. T. 1978. Ethical issues related to research involving elderly subjects. *The Gerontologist, 18*(4), 326–337.

Shearer, N., Fleury, J., and Belyea, M. 2008. An innovative approach to recruiting homebound older adults. *Journal of the American Geriatrics Society, 56*(12), 2340–2348.

Wood, F., Prout, H., Bayer, A., Duncan, D., Nuttall, J., Hood, K., and Butler, C. C. 2013. Consent, including advanced consent, of older adults to research in care homes: A qualitative study of stakeholders' views in South Wales. *Trials, 14,* 247. doi: 10.1186/1745-6215-14-247.

Wrights, A. P., Fain, C. W., Miller, M. E., Rejeski, W. J., Williamson, J. D., and Marsh, A. P. 2015. Assessing physical and cognitive function of older adults in continuing care retirement communities: Who are we recruiting? *Contemporary Clinical Trials, 40,* 159–165. doi: 10.1016/j.cct.2014.12.003.

chapter seven

Training decisions

Throughout this book, material has been provided on why older adults in CCRCs need technology training, the ways that technology training may affect the lives of residents of CCRCs, complexities and best practices for implementing training programs in CCRCs, and ways to motivate residents to participate in technology training programs. Understanding these issues is important for helping decide whether to implement a technology training program in CCRCs. The focus now shifts to decisions and considerations that should be addressed when thinking about doing the actual training for residents in CCRCs.

Conducting a needs assessment will help guide the nature of the training, identify specific skills and competencies that may be needed or wanted, and aid in the development of longer term goals of the training. It can also help determine prior skill levels, experience, and types of information and communication technologies (ICTs) used currently or in the past. This information will also help guide the appropriate procedures and materials to use as well as types of trainers needed.

Training procedures, materials, and implementation are critical components to the success of any technology program in a CCRC. In this chapter, many of the issues involved in technology training are discussed, including characteristics of CCRC populations that affect training implementation, whether to do group or individual sessions, the size of classes (if doing group training) and numbers of participants to expect, the length of training sessions, characteristics needed in trainers, and whether to use individuals internal or external to the CCRC to conduct the training programs. Some of these decisions are easy to make, whereas others require substantial research and thought. Careful consideration of each of these factors will help to ensure that the technology program is delivered in such a way that it is beneficial to all those who participate.

7.1 Uniqueness of specific CCRC populations

One of the first issues that should be considered concerns the characteristics of the residents who might be potential participants in training programs. Understanding their capabilities and limitations can help in designing an effective training program. Older adults have varying levels of cognitive, motor, and perceptual abilities. Depending upon the levels of care provided by the CCRC, there can be a quite dramatic variation in residents' physical and cognitive health status, in addition to age. Deciding whether the training will be open to all residents or to only those who are residing in specific parts of CCRCs, such as assisted living or independent living, will be a consideration. Tailoring the training to the age and health characteristics of the CCRC residents is important.

Determining whether the training will be available for those who have certain cognitive and physical limitations is a necessity. For example, it may be very difficult for residents who have severe memory issues to be able to retain training information and to be able to effectively use ICTs to enhance their lives. Even though some residents may be cognitively able to begin training, our experience indicates that during an extended training period (even 8 weeks), declines will occur for a portion of the participants that may make it more difficult for them to successfully complete the training and use the skills learned. Regular repetition of key skills will help with this issue, but trainers need to stay aware of each participant's progress and retention, suggesting attendance at extra sessions or offering more personalized assistance during the training sessions to help mitigate the effects of cognitive decline.

Physical limitations should also be taken into account. For many older adults, manual dexterity is not as good as when they were younger. This has implications for the types of ICTs to be used and whether modifications may be needed (e.g., a large trackball may be easier to use than a standard mouse). Rooms will also need to accommodate wheelchairs, canes, oxygen devices, walkers, and so forth. Chairs and table height should be comfortable for residents with a variety of physical health complaints. Extra padding may be needed in chairs to keep participants comfortable while sitting through a training session. Reducing clutter, cords, and training materials is important for decreasing fall potential. Many of these issues are discussed in greater detail in Chapter 3.

Health declines may occur over the course of the training, which may make it difficult for participants to continue training or return to training after being sick or hospitalized. Be prepared to offer personal assistance to those who may miss a few sessions due to health, offer additional assistive devices as needed, or rearrange the physical setup to accommodate returning participants. Unfortunately, there will sometimes be cases where the participant will simply be unable to continue due to physical or cognitive decline. By working closely with trainers and CCRC staff, these participants may still be able to continue to use the technology to some degree. See more in-depth coverage of these issues in Chapter 6.

Another aspect to consider is that older adults in CCRCs, especially those in independent living and those who are more mobile, may travel extensively, particularly during the winter months. Considering whether the CCRC has a significant number of "snow-birds" will help to determine the best time of the year to offer ICT training.

Our experience suggests that at times staff, and sometimes residents, of different care levels or units of a CCRC may not want to train together. In our training, this issue was more salient for CCRC staff than it was for the residents. We conducted training sessions in some communities in which the activity director of the independent living section did not want to have residents from the assisted living section involved. Sometimes, this was due to the cognitive or physical limitations of the residents. Other times, it appeared to be related to where the training activities might take place; for instance, an activity director at one site did not think that residents from assisted living would be willing to take part in a training held in independent living. She worried that the physical distance to the training site in another building where the independent living residents resided would make it difficult for residents in assisted living to participate. In reality, this did not appear to impede the participation among residents in assisted living. At times, CCRC staff may carry over experiences and attitudes from other activities when making decisions about something like a technology training program.

It was less often the case that residents did not want to mix for the training programs. When there were issues, it was normally the case that residents in independent living did not want to be in activities with residents of assisted living. They noted that residents in assisted living had more issues with frailty and impairment, which might impede the training. Even though residents may not want to mix for some activities, do not assume that this would also apply to a technology training program. However, it may be a factor that affects which groups are offered training and whether the training is held with individuals from different parts of the CCRC at the same time.

Conducting a needs assessment to help understand the uniqueness and the challenges of the residents of CCRCs will help to determine the types and functions of technology training that are needed and that can potentially be conducted successfully. Having this foundation will also help to determine the anticipated numbers of residents who might be able and wish to participate.

7.2   Anticipated numbers

Unless there is an experienced activities director who has a very good sense of which residents are likely to participate in the type and schedule of training sessions developed, estimates of the number of participants are likely to be very inaccurate. Guesses based on the number of people "who have talked about wanting a class" or the number of people "who have a computer" are not reliable indicators. The best estimate comes from a well-attended information session at which people sign up, followed by a 7- to 10-day period in which others can either sign up or ask for further information. The numbers gathered in this way are rarely off by more than two or three participants and are often very close, as some who sign up do not attend and some who did not sign up will show up the first day of class and ask if they can join. That said, there are no reliable rules for judging how many or what percentage of given population will be interested in participating.

Generally speaking, independent living residents, often being younger and in better health, tend to participate in larger numbers than do assisted living residents. Skilled care and nursing care residents may not be cognitively or physically capable of participating, depending upon the severity of the health issue. If they are able to participate, they may require more assistance with following the training procedures than will other residents.

The location of the sessions also has far less of an effect on independent living participation than it does on assisted living participation, with independent living residents being able to attend sessions in less convenient locations. As a side note, however, be aware of unspoken bias toward different potential training locations. As mentioned earlier in this chapter, some locations may carry a stigma for different groups within an assisted or independent living community, especially communities where a spectrum of continuing care is offered. For example, some independent living residents may be biased against attending sessions held in areas they perceive to be for the assisted living residents. If there are differing levels of living space available, for example, in independent living that includes free-standing houses or townhomes in addition to more traditional apartment-style units, those living in the free-standing units may be less likely to attend sessions in areas that are perceived as normally reserved for those in apartment-style units.

We will not repeat here all the ways in which different choices can affect recruitment and participation numbers, but do recall that the time of day, length of sessions, schedule, location, and topics covered will all affect how many residents are willing to enroll and attend regularly. (See Chapter 6 for more on recruitment and retention.) Whatever the interest, however, it is wise to limit the upper enrollment to around 20 participants (assuming the goal is to do group training and there is appropriate staffing). Even if there is extra staffing that will allow even larger classes, these can become unwieldy—difficult to set up, difficult for many participants to hear or see because of classroom layout and general noise, and difficult for trainers to navigate due to the number of cords, tables, and chairs needed. If interest in participation is very high, it is much better to offer separate sessions, perhaps two sets of sessions rather than one. In this case, however, it is wise to have participants commit to one or the other set of sessions so that participants do not migrate to one session or the other, causing overload. By having them commit to one set of sessions, they may also form stronger bonds with other residents who are participating in the same training sessions and feel more comfortable asking questions when they have come to know other residents.

7.3   Individual versus group training sessions

Different things are accomplished during group training sessions compared to individual training sessions. Group training sessions are much better suited to high-level, broad overview approaches, where topics or techniques are introduced and demonstrated. In these types of sessions, the instructors set the topics and pace. Very small group and individual training sessions are much better suited to hands-on practice and in-depth exploration of particular topics after basic computer training has occurred. In these types of sessions, the topics and pace are better set by the participants.

Our own experience combined these different kinds of training sessions so as to provide both broad-based experience and small group/ individual learning opportunities for participants. As noted in previous chapters, the large group sessions covered a preset range of material and included handouts, a training manual, and predefined lessons. Although there were elements of hands-on practice in these settings, it was the rare participant who found the amount of group versus hands-on work to be just right. For some participants, there was too much time for hands-on work and these participants sat bored (although patiently) or explored on their own while others received help with the tasks of the class. For others, there was not enough time for hands-on practice. As a result, these participants could sometimes feel somewhat rushed to move on to the next topic even though they felt that they could use more practice.

Although this might suggest screening for ability of participants and grouping them according to ability, we would suggest that there are advantages to having a diversity of skill levels in the same class. We encouraged those who were more skilled or who learned the training material quicker to help those who were struggling, thus encouraging the class members to rely upon each other for assistance. We were also available for assistance, but we wanted to encourage them to help each other so that they could be resources for each other when we were not onsite or available via other means.

Had the large group sessions been the only type of training offered, we probably would have had more attrition, either from frustration or from boredom. However, the office hours sessions provided an opportunity for more individualized instruction during which the frustrated participants could get one-on-one guidance to help them master the material covered during the large class. Similarly, the participants who had perhaps been bored by the pace of the larger class often found that the office hours time provided a good chance to go deeper into a topic of interest or get assistance with topics that could not be covered in the larger class.

This may seem to suggest that the best approach would be to always offer both types of sessions; however, if the group of participants is smaller and all are comparable in skills and interest, then perhaps group sessions with a great deal of hands-on free time would suffice. If, however, the same small group has participants of greatly varying skill and interest, then perhaps individual training sessions scheduled at the participant's convenience would be a better option, if staffing allows. The hybrid method we employed seems to work best for larger groups with greatly varying skills and interests.

7.4   Training duration

There are two categories of duration to consider when designing training sessions: the duration of a single session and the duration of the course. The duration of single sessions is the simpler of the two. Single sessions may vary in length, depending on whether they are group or individualized sessions. It may be tempting to keep sessions very short in order to accommodate participants' ability to sit and absorb new material for a given length of time. However, it is difficult with a group to cover very much at all in a session as short as 30 minutes, as setup and introduction of the material would consume at least half of the allotted time. If, however, individualized sessions are being conducted, 30 minutes may be sufficient, depending on the material to be covered. Sessions should not exceed about 90 minutes at the longest. Past this point, both physical and mental fatigue set in. From the instructor's perspective, 90 minutes is a good amount of time to introduce and practice a coherent module of material (e.g., writing and sending an email or setting up a social media account). In our experience, we rarely, if ever, encountered participants for whom 90 minutes was enough of an issue to preclude participation. Similarly, in office hours sessions, some participants stayed the entire 90 minutes, whereas others would come by for as little as 15–20 minutes to practice something or ask questions.

The larger question is the duration of the sessions for the course as a whole. As described in previous chapters, our prototype was an 8-week course, modified from an original 6-week design after pilot testing showed that the shorter timeframe was too rushed, given what we wanted to cover.

The consensus among participants seemed to be that the course could have been even longer, covering some topics in greater detail and expanding to cover other topics. If staffing allows and resident interest is high enough, one could imagine a rolling, continuous course in which material is revisited on a regular and continual basis, reinforcing the material for those who have already participated and introducing the material to new residents or participants. Such a design would fit well with many of the other activities often found in CCRCs, which are ongoing, with rotating content.

Our work also suggests that ongoing support is needed in order for CCRC residents to be able to continue to use ICTs over long periods of time. As noted above, some portion of participants will inevitably experience declines in physical or cognitive health during and after the training. These declines will often necessitate additional assistance to maintain skills in using ICTs. Health issues are one of the strongest factors that lead older adults in CCRCs to discontinue the use of ICTs. In addition, even for those who have not experienced health declines, our experience suggests that having support personnel available to answer questions when problems arise, updating devices, acquiring new devices, and so forth are important for CCRC residents to be able to continue to use ICTs in a meaningful way. In addition, having a short, perhaps 2 week long, refresher course about 2–3 months after the training ends may help participants maintain their skills and address areas that need additional training. It is necessary to incorporate these elements into your training decisions.

7.5   Training location

Careful consideration needs to be given to the location for the training sessions. If you are doing individual training, you will have more options. You could do the training in many open or common areas, the residents' rooms, library, and so on. However, if you plan to do group training, you will need a larger space that can accommodate the number of residents you expect to participate. This should be a topic of discussion with the CCRC staff and trainers. They may have preferences, which may or may not work well within the CCRC. By thinking about issues noted in this chapter, you should have a clear idea of the type of space that will be needed and key factors that may affect the implementation and success of the training. See Chapters 3 and 4 for a more detailed discussion on location considerations.

7.6   Who will do the training?

The default may be to turn to someone who knows a lot about technology. Although this person certainly needs to be on hand to troubleshoot and provide support, the best person to lead the training is one who is

Table 7.1 Training factors to consider

1. Who the trainers will be
2. Background and knowledge needed
3. Interpersonal characteristics
4. Number of trainers and assistants needed
5. Consistency in training personnel and methods

knowledgeable enough to cover the material in a thorough way while also being personable, calm, and patient. Although the trainer should know enough about the topics being presented to come across as well-informed and self-assured, it is more important that participants trust the trainer and feel that the trainer and the supporting staff understand them and want them to succeed. When making training decisions, there are several factors to consider (see Table 7.1).

7.6.1   Background and knowledge needed

The trainer need not be a technology expert or have experience teaching about the technology. More important is the experience and demeanor necessary to put CCRC residents at ease and provide a comfortable, non-intimidating technology learning environment. The trainer should be knowledgeable enough about the topics being covered that he or she can present the material in an authoritative, comprehensive manner and not be stumped by simple questions, get lost in the material, or be thrown off by minor technical issues. It is important that, from the participants' perspective, the trainer is well in control.

Mostly, this means experience more than expertise. If, for example, the topic is web-based email, it is more important for the trainer to have a great deal of experience with the platform being used than to have in-depth technical knowledge about email or the Web. Sufficient experience will endow the trainer with the ease necessary to present the material and provide demonstrations in a confident, easy manner that will, in turn, inspire confidence and a willingness to try on the part of the participants. Conversely, a great deal of technical knowledge, but not a lot of experience, can lead to an over-focus on minutiae and a lack of confidence when minor difficulties arise. In short, an easygoing, experienced confidence is far more important than detailed technical knowledge.

7.6.2   Interpersonal characteristics

In order to project an easygoing, experienced confidence, the primary characteristics required are interest, patience, and perseverance.

Instructing groups of older adults in technology that is unfamiliar to them can be a daunting task. On the best of days, with the most interested of participants, there is still often an underlying question of "I've gotten this far without it, so why do I need it now?" In our experience, the smallest sign of disinterest, impatience, or frustration on the part of the trainer or support staff will be noticed by participants and often taken as a sign that the people doing the training do not want to be doing it, or worse, that attempting to teach older adults about new technologies may be viewed as a lost cause. The trainer and staff must show participants that they care about the participants' success, that no amount of questioning, repetition, or misunderstanding is too much, and that the trainer and staff are there for as long as it takes to help participants learn and master what they need to be independent users of a new technology—even if the trainer and staff do not actually always feel that way.

The stereotypical "tech person" is impatient and condescending. What is needed for training in CCRCs is exactly the opposite. Rather than telling a participant to move out of the way when something goes wrong, the trainer should insist that the participant stay where she is while the trainer walks her through the steps needed to correct the problem. Rather than getting frustrated and finishing a task for a participant, the assistant should stick with him until the task is completed, reminding him along the way that the assistant understands how hard it can be to learn something new and that perhaps he or she had similar difficulties when first learning. At all times, trainers and supporting personnel should project an image of calm, caring professionalism and interest that tells participants that nothing that comes up is a problem and that they are there for as long as it takes.

To the extent that any of these factors make for a good lead trainer, the same characteristics make for good assistants, even more so. Whereas the lead trainer will mostly address the group at large (for group training sessions), the assistants are in the trenches, so to speak, where they must deal more at a one-on-one level with participants—participants who can become frustrated, misunderstand instructions, or simply fail to follow instructions or examples, often repeatedly. The key is to avoid paternalism and always, in a calm, patient, and respectful manner, guide the participants in doing tasks themselves so that the participants learn what to do and how to do it. Still, there are times when it is clear that a participant may not be capable of performing a particular task. At such times, the trainer or assistant must take special care to assist in carrying out the task without appearing paternalistic, annoyed, or frustrated.

In posttraining evaluations, the older adults we worked with cited the fact that we did not "talk down to them or treat them like they were stupid" as key to their enjoyment of and interest in the class. This led many of them to note that our training was by far the best that they had ever experienced.

It is easy for those who are doing the training to want to control the situation and fix problems so that training can continue. Our experience suggests that this is not a successful way for older adults in CCRCs to learn to use ICTs. Being supportive, caring, respecting their skills and experiences, and allowing them to "learn by doing" are critical to their success.

7.6.3   Number of trainers and assistants needed

If there is a rule of thumb that applies to staffing the types of training scenarios presented in this text, it is that you will probably need more staff than you expect. This happens for two reasons. First, the primary trainer needs to remain largely at the front of the room where he or she can demonstrate on the large screen and, for group training sessions, keep the sessions on track. If the primary trainer is always leaving the front to assist participants, you risk frustrating the other participants and causing them to lose interest. Of course, it is acceptable for the trainer to leave the front occasionally, especially during extended periods of practice on the part of participants—for example, while participants are composing an email or social media post. However, the primary trainer should always be ready and able to return to the front to demonstrate or illustrate points of technique or to answer questions. Put succinctly, do not expect your primary trainer to also walk the room as an assistant.

To determine appropriate staffing for assistants, it is wise to start with a few more than you expect to need and then cut back if appropriate. Better to start with too many and then reduce staffing, than start with too few and risk frustration on the part of participants who do not feel they are getting the help they want or need. In a similar vein, different lessons will require different levels of assistance and, therefore, more or fewer assistants. We routinely found that account creation days, days on which the class exercise was to set up email or social media accounts, required additional staff on our team, as participants routinely needed a good deal of personal attention and assistance. In contrast, days where general overviews of topics were presented (e.g., a session on the big picture of social media or evaluating health information found online) required only a couple of assistants, no matter how large the class, because the material was not as hands-on.

Given these caveats, a staff of one lead trainer and one assistant for every five participants should cover most situations. Again, however, actual staffing needs will depend largely on the health status, experience, and expectations of participants and the material being covered. For some sessions and some mixes of participants (e.g., classes with very inexperienced, timid participants), this staffing plan could be stretched thin. For other sessions and mixes of participants, you may find staffing at this level leaves people standing around without much to do. If you find that certain participants require nearly constant assistance, consider assigning one or more assistants on a permanent or rotating basis to spend most of their time with those participants. You may even consider rearranging seating to put participants who require a lot of assistance close together so that they can be assisted by fewer staff; for example, stationing one staff member between two participants who regularly need a great deal of help would be a good idea. In such cases, add to the staff rather than letting others in the session go without assistance. Regardless of the staffing level, remember to take into account setup and breakdown times with the staff you have available and allow appropriate time for both.

7.6.4 *Consistency in training personnel and methods*

Consistency in approach is perhaps more important than consistently having the same lead trainer or assistants. As mentioned earlier, having someone who is knowledgeable and experienced and who can project an air of assured confidence is very important. Developing (or procuring) a training manual or guide and staying with it is an important consideration in keeping the materials and methods consistent so that participants know what to expect from session to session and can approach them with confidence and ease.

Using the same format from session to session (e.g., introduction, recap of previous session, overview of current session, new material, practice, recap, and preview of next session) will help participants stay oriented to the sessions and material and better follow along. Having training that builds on each skill learned, reinforces skill development, and proceeds logically are important to enable older adults to acquire ICT skills. Consistency and repetition are key to successful acquisition and retention of skills for CCRC populations.

7.6.5 *Do it yourself or contract it out*

In the prior sections, we have detailed factors and characteristics that make for a good trainer. These factors and characteristics will be needed whether the training is conducted by someone working within the CCRC or someone who is part of an external organization. Deciding who will do the training is one of the key decisions that has to be made—whether the training will be done by individuals within the CCRC and/or volunteers, or whether the CCRC should contract the training activities to an outside organization. Each of these options has costs and benefits.

If there is access to appropriate internal personnel, it may be beneficial to conduct the training internally. Chances are that CCRC trainers may have had some interaction with residents and may be more comfortable working with them if they have an established relationship. Internal staff may also have a better sense of the unique characteristics of the residents in the specific CCRC and potentially be able to tailor the training to the characteristics of these residents. If the trainers are internal to the organization, they may also be more likely to be present between training sessions; given this, residents may be able to seek assistance from them at times other than during the training sessions and trainers may be able to help better integrate skills into other aspects of community life. This may benefit residents in terms of enhancing their ICT skills and being able to maintain these skills for longer periods of time.

Using trainers internal to the CCRC may also have some disadvantages. Staff may not have the skills needed to effectively train residents to use ICTs with which the staff are not familiar. As noted in this and other chapters, certain skills are needed in order to effectively train older adults, particularly those with limited ICT experience, to cross the digital divide and to be able to use ICTs effectively. Internal trainers may feel comfortable using the technology themselves but not be able to effectively communicate training steps in ways that are tailored for older adults. They may also not have adequate time to do the training, particularly if they are doing the training in addition to their existing duties.

7.6.6 External contractor decisions—How to find and evaluate external trainers

A CCRC may not have the staff and other resources to allow it to train residents in the use of particular ICTs. If this is the case, it may be wise to seek an external contractor to conduct the training. Contracting out the training is easier in some ways, particularly if there is an organization that has experience training older adults who are CCRC residents or individuals who are similar to the residents of the CCRC. In some areas of the country, there may be many potential organizations that could do training; however, in others there may be few or no such organizations. A first step is identifying the options.

One of the best and most convenient ways to find external organizations or individuals who can do ICT training is to rely on social networks. Talk with others who have worked with such entities. Chances are that staff at other CCRCs in the geographic area, senior centers, aging outreach organizations, or libraries know of those who do this type of training. Hearing their experiences with particular trainers and organizations will also be beneficial in helping decide who to use for CCRC training.

A second way to find potential training organizations is to contact local, regional, and national older adult organizations and associations (e.g., AARP, Area Agencies on Aging, Senior Services of America, and SeniorNet) to see if they have lists of individuals and organizations in the area that do this type of training. Reviewing their publications and websites may also be useful, as they may include information about potential organizations that could do the training.

If the CCRC is part of a corporate group or other association of CCRCs, staff within the CCRC network may have suggestions of organizations that could assist with training. Some of the larger chains of CCRCs are now integrating training into many of their sites. Even if the CCRC is not part of a larger network, its staff may still be able to suggest options that could be useful. Another avenue is to reach out to people in local technology organizations. They may know of different initiatives that could potentially help in training CCRC residents.

See Table 7.2 for questions that should be posed to those being considered as external trainers as well as answers that indicate a good fit. Trainers with external organizations should have experience working with older adults and be familiar with the specific challenges of working with this population. If they do not have such experience, then other options might be better. For relevant examples of challenges of working with older adults in CCRCs, see Section 7.1 of this chapter.

Outside training organizations should also have established training regimens that can be modified to meet the needs of a CCRC population. Decisions will need to be made as to the goals for the training, overall training timeframe, duration of each session, number of sessions, and the interactive nature of the training. Resources to be provided by the CCRC, as well as those by the outside vendor, will need to be specified. For instance, does the CCRC, the external vendor, or the individuals being trained provide the ICTs used for the training? Having ICTs that are similar or identical will ensure easier training in many instances. Also, what materials will be provided to trainees (e.g., training manuals, handouts, phone number to call with questions, and so on)?

Disadvantages of using external contractors include cost, coordination, and scheduling, and also potential lack of familiarity with your specific population. Although it is likely that there may be several outside vendors who could train the CCRC residents, some locales may not have outside organizations capable of conducting this type of training. Contacting local libraries and senior centers for available resources might provide an additional source of information in these situations. Considering training via webinars or other tele-hosting services might also be an option, though this would most likely not be as beneficial to successful training as would in-person training sessions.

Table 7.2 Questions for and answers by external training vendors

Questions	Answers that suggest an appropriate training vendor
What experience do you have in training older adults who are similar to residents of this type of CCRC?	Answers describe • Prior experience with CCRC communities or older adult populations in general • Prior experience with training on the use of ICTs in general and with older adults
What is the background of your trainers, and how were they trained to train others?	Answers give details about • Formal or informal education in training • Training theories that guide training • Sociodemographic characteristics and how they relate to the CCRC population of interest
Do you offer individual or group training sessions?	Answers give reasons for using various teaching methods, including • Individual (one-on-one) sessions • Small group (one-to-few) sessions • Larger group training sessions
What are your preferences for locations for training?	Answers indicate awareness of advantages and disadvantages of various training locations, including • Sites within the CCRC • External organization sites
What resources are provided and by whom?	Answers discuss who is to provide • ICTs • Written materials • Training manuals • Software • Online materials • Phone access • Trainer access outside of training sessions
What resources does the CCRC need to provide?	Answers may include • Wi-Fi • Tables and chairs • ICTs
What are the costs associated with the training you offer?	Answers give details in one or more formats, such as • Cost per person • Cost per group • Cost per session • Cost per year • Cost per hour

Table 7.3 Comparison table

Organization name	For profit (FP) versus nonprofit (NP)	Experience training in CCRCs	Group or individual training format	Materials provided by organization	Costs
Company A	FP	Yes	Both	Devices and training manuals	$ per person
Company B	NP	No	Both	Training manuals	$ per class
Individual A	NP	No	Individual	Training manuals	$ per person

If talking with more than one organization about training, we suggest making a table to keep track of responses for later comparison and decision making. An example is shown in Table 7.3. We also suggest talking with references to find out how successful the organizations' training sessions were with other populations, in other settings, and so on.

Cost may vary quite dramatically depending upon the resources provided, number of personnel involved in training, and scale of the organization. We do not offer price suggestions, given that market conditions vary considerably, depending upon regional and other factors. Keep in mind, however, that there will be some economies of scale. It will not be the case that training for five participants will be half the cost of training for 10 participants, as both require some basic level of equipment, personnel, setup, and travel.

Consider corporate, nonprofit, and volunteer options for providing training. Costs may vary depending upon the type of organization chosen. In addition, different organizations may have different philosophies in terms of teaching older adults that might relate more or less well to the CCRC population of interest.

If volunteers are preferred, conduct due diligence with them as you would with other individuals and organizations to make sure that they would be good trainers for the CCRC population. Find out their experience in this area and their willingness to commit to the full training schedule. Think about the characteristics we noted earlier in this chapter that are needed in effective trainers and discuss how they would structure training with the population of interest. There are various individuals who have been volunteering their time and energy for many years, trying to help older adults cross the digital divide. Talking with senior centers and libraries may help you identify some of these individuals in your community.

7.7   Fit with CCRC population

Although we have touched upon this issue before in this and earlier chapters, we think it wise to reiterate it again here. Regardless of whether using a corporate, nonprofit, volunteer, or other option for training residents, consider the fit with the CCRC population. If the trainers do not understand the challenges and the positive benefits of working with older adults, many of whom may have specific health challenges, the training may not be successful. Make sure that the individual or organization that is chosen understands the unique characteristics of the population that resides in the CCRC.

In summary, this chapter has provided an overview of key decisions that need to be made regarding training and trainers before implementing a technology training program in CCRCs. Although many considerations need to be taken into account, thinking through these issues should provide adequate guidance to determine whether the training can be done by CCRC staff or whether an external individual or organization should conduct the training.

Recommended readings

Czaja, S. and Sharit, J. 2013. *Designing training and instructional programs for older adults.* Boca Raton, Florida: CRC Press.

Rogers, W. A., Campbell, R. H., and Pak, R. 2001. A systems approach for training older adults to use technology. In N. Charness, D. C. Parks, and B. A. Sabel (Eds.), *Communication, technology and aging—Opportunities and challenges for the future* (pp. 187–208). New York: Springer.

Swezey, R. W. and Llaneras, R. E. 1997. Models in training and instruction. In G. Salvendy (Ed.), *Handbook of human factors and ergonomics* (2nd ed., pp. 514–577). New York: Wiley.

chapter eight

Current needs for technological access and use in continuing care retirement communities

Learning how to use technology, like learning any new skill, requires continued support and practice. Because of technology's ever-changing nature, the skills one learns must be continually updated. For older adults, this can be quite frustrating and can impede the continued use of technology. The skills they initially learn will have to be changed and adjusted for each new technology or each new update of their current technology. Something as simple as changes in the interface of the email system can throw off their usage patterns due to frustration and irritation. To overcome some of these issues, we tried to anticipate changes in the interface, issues with access, and the need for continual support. By anticipating issues in these areas and trying to incorporate new avenues of use through pulling in family members, we hoped to find ways to keep older adults engaged with the technology longer. This chapter addresses how we anticipated these needs and addressed these issues.

8.1 Interface

Coverage of topics such as interface design and the science of human interaction with technology is beyond the scope of this book, but the Recommended Readings section at the end of this chapter lists sources specific to design for older adults. However, our experience with technology training using computers, the Internet, and, in a limited way, tablets has provided insights into the importance of good interface design for older adults. That said, the ideas discussed here concern a rapidly changing field. As today's younger people become tomorrow's older adults, the specifics of interface considerations will surely change. Nonetheless, some overarching considerations will likely remain.

One thing that became readily apparent when we began our technology training sessions was that the very common paradigm of the Microsoft Windows® operating system was not familiar to most of the older adults in the CCRCs in which we worked. The same was true for the now entrenched paradigm behind the presentation of most Web pages within Web browsers. The pointing, clicking, right-clicking, scrolling, and so on that most users take for granted in any computer interface were strange and different to most of our older adult students. Browsing files and folders, following links, and performing tasks such as typing a search term into a text box were likewise strange to older adults. Vocabulary as simple as "click" or "move the mouse" often took more than one class to master. Although we anticipated that this would be the case and took account of it in our planning and training materials, it was still a stark realization when the training started.

Although a few of the older adult students continued to struggle with the interface, most were able to master it fairly quickly. This process was aided by the use of simplified terminology in the training manual; repetitive, detailed instructions; and repetitive practice for even the most simple of tasks (e.g., opening a program). Although we had limited experience with older adults and the use of tablets (some participants in our trainings would bring their tablets to our office hours sessions), we found that the touch interface was much simpler for older adults to understand and use. It removed the extra layer of moving a mouse and clicking a button. Pointing and touching with a finger did not require a shift in thinking. Using touch screens made more sense to them than using the point-and-click method.

This difference between touching and pointing and clicking highlights the larger lesson learned through our training experiences. Although interfaces and interactive paradigms can and will change with changing technologies, the important thing for those working with older adults and technology to remember is that the simpler the interface can be made, whether by design or through the way the instructor explains and teaches it, and the less removed from actual physical experience (e.g., touch, rather than point and click), the easier it will be for those unfamiliar with it to grasp and master. Therefore, no matter the interface or how technology advances, the main goal of design should be naturalization and simplification, both of which take a great deal of thought and time to effectively implement in training. Although this may be less of a problem in the future, the necessity for a simple and natural interface will continue for at least the next decade.

Pilot testing the training materials and curriculum is crucial. For example, one difficulty that we did not anticipate through our months of preparation and planning was that it would be difficult for some participants to understand the concept of holding the mouse still while clicking. Many of our older adult users had great difficulty with this, often moving the mouse ever-so-slightly when pressing the button to click. We were able to overcome this issue for many people by having them use either a trackball or track pad, separating the mechanics of pointing from the mechanics of clicking. However, the track pads offered a different layer of complexity for those who might not have complete sensation in their fingers or who have extreme arthritis. Although giving multiple options might be easier, it creates a learner hierarchy within the group and some will feel as if it is a competition to use the most "normal" method even when it is more difficult for them. Therefore, it is important to try to naturalize and simplify as many aspects as possible for the learner.

8.2   Access

When we started our training sessions, access to ICTs in most CCRCs we worked with was extremely limited. In communities that did happen to have a shared computer, for example, in a library, it was often a very old computer without access to the Internet. Some residents had their own Internet access, but it might have been set up by a well-meaning relative who was no longer around to provide the support needed for the resident to make good use of it. By the end of our training sessions, several CCRCs were installing Wi-Fi systems for residents' use. Still, there was often little support for the residents if they had trouble getting connected, staying connected, or otherwise using the system. The information technology providers for the communities often had a difficult time discussing issues with connection or usage on a simple level for new users.

Even as physical access improves, whether through better infrastructure or better provision of workstations, laptops, or tablets, access without adequate support can be worse than no access at all, causing confusion and frustration. Providing access is the easy part of the equation. Creating a supportive culture and environment is far more difficult and labor intensive, and requires a greater commitment on the part of CCRC management and staff. As ICTs, Wi-Fi, and the Internet become even more pervasive, it is not uncommon for CCRCs to tout the quality and amount of access they provide as amenities that set their locations apart from those of their competitors. In our view, what truly distinguishes locations that are doing an excellent job is not the amount of access provided, but rather the provision of the support necessary to take full advantage of whatever access is provided. Although CCRC staff may occasionally be able to answer a question or troubleshoot a problem, it is important to have dedicated personnel who can assist residents or offer a type of "continuing education" training. Having toll-free numbers to call when one is having trouble is no substitute for an in-person troubleshooter who can demonstrate to the resident how to fix many of his or her own problems and make better use of his or her technology. Anyone can install Wi-Fi routers to cover an entire community. Ensuring that residents have the support and encouragement needed to make good use of that technology is the true measure of access.

8.3   Keep it simple

The primary point we take from our experience and reading on these topics is keep it simple. This means not only designing and implementing simple, easy-to-use interfaces or technology, but also designing training interventions and support services to bridge the gap when the interfaces and technology are not as simple as they could be. This mostly means making interaction with technology as natural as possible. As said earlier in this chapter, using the point-and-touch method is much more natural than using the point-and-click method. It may also mean the mechanical separation of tasks—for example, separating pointing from clicking, so that it is no longer point *and* click, but point *then* click.

Keeping it simple also means avoiding the unnecessary complexity of unneeded detail. One need not know how a computer works to make good use of the Internet to communicate with loved ones and research topics of interest. Whereas people who work with computers as a hobby may revel in the details of workings of the computer, most older adults will do much better with interfaces and technologies that hide as much of the computer as possible, eschewing esoteric metaphors such as file systems and desktops in favor of configurations such as cloud-based systems where documents, pictures, and the like are simply always available from any device. To paraphrase Steve Jobs, go for the systems that "just work" without a lot of tinkering, maintenance, or need for detailed knowledge about how they function. Put simply, when working with older adults in CCRCs, move as much of the complexity and detail as possible behind the curtain, either through the use of the well-designed interfaces and technology or through well-designed training that cuts away the muddling detail.

8.4   Continual support

Have you ever tried to learn a foreign language? How much did you rely on conversations with others to accomplish that goal? When you no longer had a way to interact with someone to speak the language, was it still easy to remember and to advance? Technology can be a new language to many older adults. They need people to reach out to for continued support. Anticipating this problem, we tried to locate resident experts in each community. When we located these experts, we asked if they would be willing to serve their community for any questions that might arise. We made sure to tell them they were not expected to know every answer—they were [only] there to talk through issues with or provide simple reminders about basic technological tasks. If they agreed, then they were identified to the class before the end of the training. During our training sessions, we found that many times our participants simply wanted someone to sit with them and affirm their choices until they felt they clearly knew the tasks. The community-based experts served this function after the initial training was over. This provided an additional level of support for participants and an ability for the communities to form interest groups to continue their learning.

When selecting these experts, we found that it was just as important to select for personality as it was to select for skill. If the individual was not up for the job or found it too overwhelming, then it was not useful to the community. However, once identified, most were happy to oblige. Many really felt that it was an honor and enjoyed the new title. It gave them an additional purpose in the community.

After each training session was complete, office hours were held for an additional month to catch any major issues or questions that arose. Additionally, throughout the training, participants had the ability to call research staff for assistance during normal business hours. They could also leave messages at other times and have someone return their calls during normal business hours. These calls could be about anything they learned that week or something that the individual had an interest in learning. The trainers were taught how to give simple, step-by-step instructions to the participant. Although most participants did not utilize this service, knowing it was there was reassuring to many. They were more willing to try something they were not sure of because if a problem arose, they knew they would be able to call someone for help with the issue. It is important to encourage the older adults to have telephone access when working at the computer so that they can easily call for help if they encounter a problem.

It was also important to residents that their ability to learn and use the technology was affirmed, even if it took a little longer to pick up new concepts. Training programs should include a repudiation of stereotypes of older adults and technology use prevalent in mass media. Some of our participants were apologetic when they were unable to quickly learn and use a new concept. They expressed a sense of embarrassment that they had little or no knowledge of how to even turn a computer on.

Although not implemented in our training, creating interest groups or reaching out to high schools, religious groups, and so forth for additional support after the initial training would be useful. This continued support, even if sporadic, would help keep the conversation going around the use of ICTs in CCRCs.

8.5   *The importance of outsiders for continued use*

Much like the importance of keeping the conversation going about technology to ensure continued use, incorporating families and friends of the user into their technology use is important. Many older adults reported that the only reason they had an interest in learning was to help connect them with their friends and family. It was an additional way to maintain contact with people who were important to them. They saw it as a noninvasive means of sending their children, grandchildren, and others messages. Many saw technology use as providing another link to their family through using social media sites. For some, technology training simply provided context for a conversation topic that they would now better understand. In our project, many of the residents liked being able to stay in communication with faith-based organizations. Receiving their organization's newsletter or weekly updates made them feel more connected even if they were unable to attend services.

Throughout the project, we attempted to find ways to engage the participants with the technology. Initially, we thought incorporating school children as email pen pals would help older adults hone their skills on email and create new intergenerational partnerships. However, this idea gained little traction. Due to barriers with how the children were able to contact the residents, one email with a long list of questions was typically sent to our trainers, who then had to facilitate the participants' answering the questions during class time. Given the lack of typing skills of the majority of the participants in our training sessions, responding to the long series of questions through typing was burdensome and task intensive for most of them. Others may find alternative ways to format such an interaction, perhaps through Skype or FaceTime, which might be easier for older adults to participate in without overburdening them.

The older adult participants really wanted to communicate with their own children, grandchildren, and friends. Their communication patterns were distinctly different in email and social network communications. They did not want to share the same information they would on a phone call. Many enjoyed simple humorous emails that their families and friends would forward or short simple emails to say hello. Often it was just as important to explain the social norms around the technology as it was to explain the technology. Knowing not only the basic use and terminology but also some of the embedded social cues allowed users to feel more connected to the larger world.

Technology will continue to evolve, and new generations of older adults will continue to need tailored training programs to adapt to these changes. Ease of use, portability, and an understanding of the benefits of technology can serve as an encouragement to use technology. Most importantly, keeping the interface simple, providing easy access, integrating multiple levels of assistance in use, and connecting friends and family to the technology will ensure that these generations will continue to be able to gain benefits from the technologies that proliferate in our world.

On the basis of our experiences, we recommend:

- Understand that access is about more than just Internet access. Having ICTs that are working and easy to use is also important.
- Keep the interface design and the training simple.
- Avoid too much talk about the inner workings and hardware associated with computers.
- Encourage participants to have access to a phone when they are using the computers when trainers are not onsite.
- Be cognizant of the typing abilities of residents and whether this impedes their use of the technology.
- Use friends, family members, and religious and community organizations to provide communication partners for CCRC residents.

Recommended readings

Fisk, A. D., Rogers, W. A., Charness, N., Czaja, S. J., and Sharit, J. 2009. *Designing for older adults: Principles and creative human factors approaches* (2nd ed.). Boca Raton, Florida: CRC Press.

Pak, R. and McLaughlin, A. C. 2010. *Designing displays for older adults.* Boca Raton, Florida: CRC Press.

chapter nine

The future of technology use among older adults in continuing care retirement communities

9.1 Developments in the world of technology

In the Academy Award-nominated 2002 film *Minority Report*, Tom Cruise plays a leader in a special division of a fictional Washington, DC, police force called PreCrime in the year 2054. The film paints a picture of a technologically advanced American society that uses a variety of (at the time) fictional gadgets to fight crime and to accomplish simple everyday tasks. A striking image from the film comes toward the beginning, with Tom Cruise's Captain John Anderton standing in front of a large computer screen. The screen Anderton is viewing contains a series of images that provide clues to a crime about to be committed, and he is cycling through the images trying to find anything that can point him in the direction of where the crime will take place so that his team can swoop in and prevent it. But what is striking about the image is that Anderton is not using a keyboard and mouse to navigate through the pictures on the computer screen; instead, he is using his *hands* to signal to the computer when he wants to switch the images on the screen, zoom in, or zoom out. The computer uses spatial-recognition software to *read what Anderton's hands are doing*—with a sweeping hand movement from left to right, he can move images to the side, and with a flick of the wrist, he can turn an image.

When the film first debuted, a technology such as this was novel—it had never been seen before and existed only in the imaginations of scientists. Telling a computer what you wanted it to do *without a keyboard or a mouse*! Like much of the other technologies highlighted in the film, such a thing seemed possible only in science fiction (emphasis on "fiction"). But fast-forward to today, and such a technology seems less impossible. Most personal computers have a built-in camera that, although typically used specifically for teleconferencing, could be used for giving spatial-recognition-based instructions in the near future. Many gaming systems now incorporate cameras that can follow what the user is physically doing, giving the user the ability to use his or her own body parts to instruct the system rather than using a keyboard or a handheld controller (this feature is especially popular in sports and dancing-themed videogames). We see a version of the *Minority Report* software used in many TV shows. Even if personal computers are not yet capable of easily mimicking the spatial recognition shown in *Minority Report*, the use of a keyboard and mouse is no longer required for many devices—computers can now have touch-based screens so that users need only to touch the computer screen to give commands such as opening or closing programs. Touch-screen interfaces are especially prevalent in smartphone technologies and tablet computers.

The past few decades have produced a number of films that feature fictional technologies that, although at the time seemed impossible to manufacture, have become a reality and are commonplace. The 1999 Academy Award-winning film *The Matrix* focuses on a society trapped in a virtual world, its inhabitants being unaware that they are in a simulation; today, various online communities and games allow individuals to create avatars and live fictional lives on the Internet, similar to the scenario shown in *The Matrix* (minus the evil robots, of course). The 2008 action film *Eagle Eye* features a rogue artificial intelligence that is able to monitor the every movement of the film's characters by using a sophisticated tracking technology and hacking into cameras; today, nearly all handheld devices come with some version of GPS that allows for such tracking (and proves especially helpful when you are lost and in need of directions!). And in the Academy Award-winning 2013 romance *Her*, a man develops a romantic relationship with a conscious computer operating system; although no technology has yet been developed that mirrors such an advanced and sophisticated artificial intelligence, there exist devices and gadgets designed to provoke an emotional response in users (an example being robots made to look like animals that people may use as pets). These films, when they debuted, featured devices, tools, and alternative realities that seemed improbable—but very quickly, the ideas and technologies they used have become a reality. Perhaps, it is a bit of a cliché, but it is true: the future is now.

The emphasis of the previous chapters has been on basic Internet-connected devices (namely, computers) and how to implement training programs in CCRC settings to teach older residents to successfully use these devices. However, technology goes well beyond just Internet-connected desktop and laptop computers. What exactly does the future hold with regard to technology, and what sort of effects can it have on the residents of CCRCs? There are many exciting developments in the world of technology that offer unique and advantageous features for residents in CCRCs, and the outlook will improve as technology is continually being developed and constantly evolving. This chapter describes only a small sample of the potential new technologies being developed for older adults, and those in CCRCs more specifically (and at the rate technology has been improving over the past decade, it could be that the "future" described in this chapter will be out of date in a matter of a few short years!). This chapter also discusses potential issues associated with some of these "improvements."

9.2   What's for dinner? The inTRAnet in independent and assisted living communities

What do you do when you want to go out with friends or family for a nice meal? Chances are that if you are feeling adventurous and in the mood for trying something new, you may suggest going to a restaurant you have never been to before. But how do you know if you and your guests will like the restaurant? Of course you can check for reviews of the restaurant or ask others about their experiences there—but a good starting point may be to check the menu to see if the food offered sounds good. Many restaurants post their menus online for easy viewing to attract potential customers. Similarly, many CCRCs post their dining hall menus online so that residents can take note of the food being offered on a given day (and can thus plan their meals more easily), and it also allows the residents' families to know what they are eating and may attract (and prove to be a selling point for) people looking to move into a CCRC. Posting menus provides a convenience to residents.

However, the benefits of such postings will be realized only if residents know how to use the Internet and can navigate to the menu. Such a task may prove especially difficult for those with little to no computer experience, as navigating to the menu requires multiple steps and skills: turning on a computer, mastery of a keyboard and mouse, being able to get online, using a search bar to navigate to the official CCRC website, and using computer menus and tabs to find the meal menu on the CCRC site. For the computer savvy, this is a straightforward process; for the inexperienced, this can prove incredibly taxing. In previous chapters of this book, we outlined tips and suggestions instructors can use to teach CCRC residents to better accomplish these tasks; an alternative, however, could be to implement an *intranet* system into the community for residents to use to more easily access menus and other CCRC information.

Prior to discussing how an intranet presence can affect CCRC communities, it is important to differentiate between the Internet and intranet. Despite sounding similar, the two terms refer to very different systems. The *Internet* represents a network of connected computers that allows for the flow of communication and information across a variety of connected devices, such as computers, smartphones, and tablets. When we refer to the Internet, it is assumed that we are talking about a global network—a person using the Internet in California can communicate with a neighbor across the street, or with a family member in New York, or with a stranger in Australia. But whereas the Internet refers to a global network of connected devices, the term "intranet" is much more restrictive; it instead refers to a connected set of devices of a private group or organization. With an intranet, individuals using connected devices can only communicate with others who are also connected via the intranet. Whereas the Internet is public, an intranet is typically thought of as private.

Many employers use some form of an intranet to make sure that communication between employees remains confidential. As an example, people who work within healthcare often use an intranet so that doctors and nurses may communicate with one another about the specifics of a patient's treatment without risking that information being out on the open Web. Confidentiality is a key reason that many organizations restrict communication to an intranet. But another important reason many organizations may use an intranet is that employees have a much more streamlined computer system through which to share information. Consider email as an example. If someone wanted to send an email using the Internet, he or she could do so using a variety of different email clients (Google, Yahoo, Microsoft Office, to name but a few) and a person could receive an email from a variety of different accounts created using any (or all) of those clients. On an intranet, however, everyone would use the same email client, making communication easier and more straightforward. On an intranet, usually there are only a handful of programs, websites, and applications at a user's disposal. Only certain activities can be done, and only certain people can be contacted; but despite (or because of) these restrictions, communication and information sharing can be easier and more efficient. There is less freedom, but those on the intranet can accomplish tasks more quickly and be more productive.

So why talk about an intranet in CCRC communities at all if we typically see it used in employer–employee settings? After all, CCRC residents do not work for the communities they live in. Even so, there is a move toward incorporating an intranet into many of these communities specifically for residents and staff to be able to communicate with one another. Let us go back to the example of searching for a menu online. A resident who wanted to use the Internet to find out what was for dinner at the CCRC on a particular night would have to use a variety of skills to navigate to the correct website and find the menu. If, however, a resident wanted to use a CCRC-restricted intranet, it could be that the menu is much more readily available and easier to view. An intranet system can be designed to have an icon on a computer home screen that links specifically to the menu for the day. A resident would not have to use a search bar to find the CCRC official website nor would he or she have to wade through the site's links and tabs to find the correct webpage; all the resident would have to do is to click on the intranet link and he or she would be right at the day's menu.

Intranet systems can be specifically designed to accommodate the various needs of residents and staff. An email system or an instant-messaging application can be incorporated so that residents and staff can easily communicate with one another. An alert system can be incorporated so that residents can call for help should they or a neighbor be in trouble (e.g., if a neighbor experiences a fall). Links can be installed into the computer home screen so that residents can easily access frequently used applications such as a world news application, a weather application, or even a health encyclopedia with reliable health information (thus putting less pressure on residents to not only find but also evaluate health information found on the Internet). Finally, in addition to dining hall menus, other CCRC information can be made readily available so that residents do not have to go to the Internet to find it: for example, telephone numbers for medical personnel, maps of the community, staff biographies and credentials, and a list of activities and their times and locations for the month. The implementation of an intranet means that residents may not be able to accomplish as much compared to other systems because there would be restrictions; however, many intranet systems do allow users to still access the Internet if need be, so more computer-savvy residents could still go surf the Web if they wished.

The immediate and apparent downside of an intranet system is that it requires specific tailoring to the community and the residents; because an intranet is designed to be efficient and easy to use for certain groups, no one system is applicable across all CCRCs. CCRCs must work with computer programmers to develop a system that caters to the needs of the facility, an endeavor that in the short term can prove costly both in time and in money. The long-term benefits, however, can outweigh these costs because a successfully implemented system can potentially promote the well-being of residents, make residents' lives happier and less stressful, and provide tools for staff to administer better care.

In our training program, we actually had one community ask us *not* to come in and do an information and communication technology (ICT) intervention because they were implementing their own intranet. Their reasoning was that because their new intranet system would look vastly different from a typical computer, having two separate trainings (one for basic ICT use and one for their new system) might prove confusing to residents, especially those who had never used a computer before. Thus, rather than have us come in to do the ICT training, they held their own training interventions focused specifically on the intranet that they had installed.

If a CCRC opts to use an intranet system in the community rather than a more typical Internet-connected system, many of the principles outlined in the book (regarding the tailoring of training) will apply. However, trainers may have the added burden of assisting with the development of the intranet or in the learning of it themselves. Such obstacles should be planned for prior to scheduling an intranet-training program.

9.3   Virtual healthcare

An emerging trend in healthcare is that of *virtual healthcare*. Virtual healthcare puts a new spin on the doctor–patient relationship and changes the way in which individuals can receive diagnoses and treatments: rather than visiting a doctor's office, patients can use ICTs to contact and communicate with doctors from the comfort of their own homes to receive medical help. The use of technologies to relay medical information from one site to another for the purposes of healthcare delivery or health education is also sometimes referred to as "telehealth" or "telemedicine." For the purposes of this section, we will continue to use the term "virtual healthcare."

9.3.1   Healthcare via teleconferencing or videoconferencing

The most popular avenue through which virtual healthcare is used is teleconferencing or videoconferencing. This modality features a two-way interaction between a clinician and a patient via a live audio or audio-visual technology. Teleconferencing has increased in popularity due to the rise of services and "apps" such as Skype or FaceTime, computer programs that allow for video phone calls between Internet-connected devices. Some CCRC residents may already have these programs downloaded onto their personal computers or smartphones. Programs such as Skype and FaceTime can be especially exciting for older adults in CCRCs because they provide a means for facility-bound residents to get in touch with friends and family who may live far away and whom they may not be able to see regularly or easily. Using the microphone and camera installed in the computer or smartphone, CCRC residents get to talk to and see their loved ones on a computer or device screen. Being able to communicate with friends and family can help promote psychological well-being and overall quality of life for residents because they may feel less lonely and more connected with their family and friends through the use of these applications.

The teleconferencing devices and applications often used by healthcare professionals in visiting with patients and delivering healthcare remotely are similar to popular products such as Skype and FaceTime in that they allow for two-way communication; however, virtual healthcare typically entails a wide variety of additional features that enhance doctor–patient interaction. As an example, there are an increasing number of medical devices that can plug directly into a computer or mobile phone so that a doctor may assess vital signs of a patient remotely. Consider a CCRC resident who is in need of a routine checkup; however, due to circumstances (such as a lack of transportation), the resident cannot get to the doctor's office. If the CCRC has the necessary equipment, it is possible that the resident can go to an Internet-connected computer and, using the plugged-in vital signs monitoring device, get a measure of temperature and blood pressure, and even record self-assessed measurements of pain; because this device is connected to an Internet-enabled computer, the information can automatically be sent to the doctor, who can then use it to assess the resident's health and recommend management techniques and potential lifestyle changes. The use of devices such as a vital signs monitor to collect and transmit health data is often referred to as "remote patient monitoring."

An advantage of virtual healthcare is that the technologies used need not be restricted to doctor–patient interactions, but can be opened up for use between patients and caregivers, caregivers and doctors, patients and social workers, and so forth. An example can be seen in a study conducted by Czaja and colleagues (Czaja et al., 2013) that evaluated the use of a video-based intervention wherein videophones were installed in the home of dementia caregivers that provided tips in caregiving and allowed for video conferencing between caregivers and interventionists as well as between caregivers and other caregivers. Technologies like these, when designed properly with the needs of the user taken into careful consideration, can be easy to use and provide a number of benefits. In the case of the intervention study, Czaja and colleagues found that videophone use by their study group (which consisted mostly of caregivers with lower socioeconomic status and limited technology experience) helped alleviate caregiver distress. Despite the limited technology experience of the participants in this study, Czaja and colleagues also found that the caregivers found the videophone relatively easy to use. As with any technology, ease of use will be important for both CCRC residents and others, such as caregivers, who may also have need to use it.

9.3.2   Mobile health applications

An emerging field within the realm of health and healthcare is that of *mobile health* (or as it is more commonly known, mHealth). mHealth, as defined by the Center for Connected Health Policy (n.d.) is "health care and public health practice and education supported by mobile communication devices such as cell phones, tablet computers, and PDAs." mHealth is a distinct subcategory within virtual healthcare due to the specific use of mobile devices; because mobile technologies such as smartphones have rapidly increased in prevalence and popularity within the past few years, mHealth applications have also rapidly increased in number and in scope.

The number of mHealth applications available and in development, and the number of topics and illnesses these mHealth applications target, is exponentially increasing. It is beyond the purview of this chapter to list them all (and, in fact, an entire book can be devoted just to mHealth), but here is a sample of the types of services available through the use of mobile technologies in promoting health and healthcare that may be most applicable for older adults:

- Use of mobile technologies for the purposes of *virtual healthcare* (i.e., using a communication application to contact and communicate with a healthcare provider)
- Use of mobile technology applications in the *management of chronic health issues* (e.g., using a diet-tracker and meal-planner app to manage weight, combat obesity, or control diabetes)
- *Emergency response systems* app that allows for the user to call for help with the touch of a button in the event of an emergency
- Applications that can be used to assist with *medication adherence*, such as a smartphone app that reminds the user when to take certain pills
- *Mobile learning* applications that provide information to the general public on a series of health issues, diseases, and healthcare options
- *Health promotion* applications that allow for individuals and communities to organize and combat public health crises (e.g., a community creating an app that educates members on the risk and transmission of HIV–AIDS and provides information on prevention, testing, and treatment)

The advantages of mHealth and, more generally, virtual healthcare are clear: for populations in which travel to a doctor or other healthcare professional is difficult (due to geographic location, inability to drive, lack of alternative transportation methods, and so on), virtual healthcare provides a means for the patient to receive care in the comfort of their own home. Such technologies have been shown to significantly improve clinical care outcomes (for a review, see the American Telemedicine Association [2015]) and therefore can be incredibly advantageous to CCRC residents. These technologies may also be appealing to the CCRC itself, as virtual healthcare has been shown to be a cost-effective alternative to in-person interactions, although the amount of money saved differs based on what applications and devices are being used. Nevertheless, virtual healthcare technologies may be a strong investment for CCRCs to consider because they can help improve the health of residents and potentially save the CCRC money in the long term.

9.4   Increased access and the importance of broadband

Older adults are at a risk of decreased use of technologies and thus may not be able to reap their full benefits. The number of barriers to technology adoption and use is large, but access has always been an issue for older age groups. Older adults with little to no technology experience may lack the necessary know-how to use certain technologies, the necessary knowledge to determine whether and when they need to use the technology, the monetary resources to purchase certain devices or subscribe to online-based services, or the ability (e.g., cognitive ability) or resources (e.g., monetary funds, technology support) to learn to use new technologies. However, as we have noted previously, access to these technologies is changing, as greater numbers of older adults are going online and successfully using ICTs.

Although access to Internet-connected devices is growing, not all access is the same. The speed at which an individual can get online and send or retrieve information can have a significant effect on the types of things accessed online as well as can have a significant effect on how those things are used in everyday life—many websites and applications are designed with a high-speed Internet connection in mind, and thus these websites and applications may not load or function properly if an individual tries to navigate to them or use them with a slow Internet connection.

The traditional method for individuals to access the Internet was once through a *dial-up* connection, which used a telephone line. In recent years, a new type of access has emerged through *broadband* Internet access, which does not require the use of a telephone line and which is much faster than dial-up. Broadband Internet connections provide a higher speed of data transmission and thus allow the user to access websites and applications that are of higher quality and that require a large amount of data transmission. An example of an application that needs a large amount of data transmission is teleconferencing. The use of programs such as Skype and FaceTime requires a large amount of audio and visual data to be transmitted between devices, necessitating a faster Internet connection through broadband (such programs could not be used on a dial-up connection). Broadband allows for such services as faster website loading, streaming video, and advanced video and animation graphics, to name but a few.

Indeed, in our rapidly evolving technology-based society, broadband Internet connections are almost required in order for individuals to be able to conduct their daily business online. A recent Pew report (Horrigan and Duggan, 2015) found that Americans who do not use broadband Internet connections are "increasingly likely to view lack of broadband as a disadvantage in key areas of life." Between 2010 and 2015, the percentage of Americans who did not use broadband and who indicated that not using broadband was a major disadvantage in finding out about job opportunities and gaining new career skills rose from 36% to 43%. In the same timeframe, the percentage of Americans who did not use broadband and who indicated that this was a disadvantage rose with regard to other topics as well, including the following:

- Learning about or accessing government services (rose from 25% to 40%)
- Learning new things that may improve or enrich their lives (rose from 23% to 37%)
- Getting health information (rose from 27% to 38%)
- Keeping up with news and information (rose from 16% to 32%)

With the advantages of having a broadband connection and with the American public recognizing its increased importance, why are some populations still using a slower dial-up connection? As discussed in the previous section, access is an issue that prevents some from being able to use broadband. For individuals in rural areas, broadband may not be available. And those in lower socioeconomic brackets (i.e., poorer individuals and families) may not be able to afford a faster Internet connection even if it was available. Yet, in the case of older adults (a population that is also more likely than others to have dial-up rather than broadband), not all live in the rural countryside nor are all poor. Then why are many older adults still using dial-up connections?

Competence and confidence in technology use may be a key factor in why some older adults opt not to use broadband. As frequently cited throughout this book, older adults, particularly those with little to no technology experience, are not always quick to try new technologies or learn new technologies; they may wish to devote cognitive efforts to other activities or may be under the impression that they are "too old" to learn something new. The flexibility of information gathering, communication, and activities provided by a broadband connection may be overwhelming to older adults just getting started with using the Internet, and they may prefer a slower connection because it restricts them to the bare basics and bare essentials of what they need to do online. Or they may not be aware of the distinctions between dial-up and broadband connections.

Expanding on this idea, Lelia Green (2010) proposes that

> People prioritise the things that are important to them ... until and unless they see a reason to want to do something else with the internet, such as watching television programmes that they have missed, which broadcasters are increasingly making possible, they are content with the level of service provided by dial-up. (p. 74)

An example Green brings up is that of email, an Internet application that is "well-serviced by dial-up." Most older adults who use the Internet use it primarily for communication purposes via email with friends and family; because email does not necessarily require a broadband connection, those older adults who use the Internet just for the purposes of email may refrain from devoting the cost and the cognitive effort to learn broadband when they can stick with what they know.

Despite what the preferences of an individual older adult may be, a CCRC looking to advance the technology capabilities of their community as well as teach its residents how to best use those technologies would do well to consider the implementation of broadband Internet and to implement a training program designed with broadband as the default and assumed connection speed (see Figure 9.1). Although some services, such

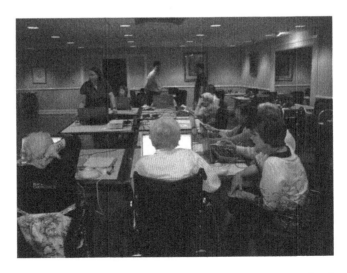

Figure 9.1 Photo from a technology training session using a wireless broadband Internet connection.

as email, do not require broadband connectivity, many others (such as teleconferencing or the use of online health websites) do.

9.5   Changing interfaces

An important consideration that ICT (and other technology) trainers need to take into account is the development and proliferation of new interfaces. For our purposes, when we refer to "interfaces," we are referring to the more general use of the term in everyday language—the parts of an ICT a user uses to communicate with the operating system of the ICT. Parts of the interface, under this definition, include the equipment such as the mouse and keyboard as well as the menus, icons, and windows the user navigates when using different computer programs. Interfaces are constantly being updated; they are streamlined to be more user-friendly, they are made more visually appealing, and new and exciting features are added so that the user can accomplish more. The constant updating of user interfaces can be a good thing, but it also poses a problem for ICT trainers, namely: are the classes and training materials applicable across old *and* new interfaces, or do these things need to be constantly amended every time the interface changes?

The good news is that for some parts of the interface, changes tend to be minimal and do not affect the training at all. This is the most apparent with external equipment such as a keyboard and mouse. Although different technology companies produce different styles of keyboards and mice (with different color schemes, different sizes, and so on), the general use of this equipment is consistent across all interfaces. All keyboards pretty much operate the same way, all traditional mice work similarly, all rollerball mice work like each other, and all touchpad mice work similarly. A well-designed technology class and a well-written training manual will be able to teach older CCRC residents to use this equipment in such a way that, if they are presented with a new set of equipment produced from a different technology company, they will still be able to use it with relative ease.

The external equipment can be an easy part of the interface to teach even with changes and updates, but the parts of the interface a user interacts with on a screen (e.g., menus, icons, and applications) can be a bit more difficult when there are changes. To illustrate this, we present a case study from one of our training classes.

9.5.1   The trouble with going from Windows Vista to Windows 8

As a reminder, in our ICT classes, we taught older adults in CCRCs to use computers and the Internet utilizing Sony Vaio laptop computers that had

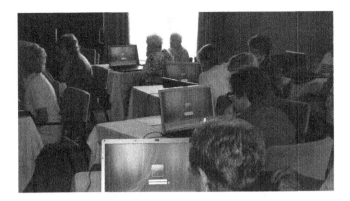

Figure 9.2 Study participants logging onto their computers, which are running the Windows Vista operating system.

the Windows Vista operating system installed (see Figure 9.2). At the start of our study in 2009, Windows Vista was a widely used operating system, and thus we felt comfortable in teaching residents to use this system— given that it was a system they might encounter elsewhere, such as on the computers of friends or family—as well as constructing a training manual that, in our mind, would likely not need much updating over the course of the study (as we did not anticipate switching to a different operating system). Like previous Microsoft operating systems, Windows Vista was simple to use. At the bottom left-hand corner of the computer screen, there was an icon that represented the Start button; by clicking on this icon (which usually just looked like a button with the Microsoft emblem in the middle), a menu (the Start menu) would open at the bottom left-hand corner of the screen with a list of programs and folders. From this menu, a person could access almost anything the computer had to offer.

Because of the ability for a user to access a computer's programs through the use of the Start button and Start menu, we emphasized the importance of the Start button in every class in our training sessions (see Figure 9.3). We spent a lot of time and effort teaching the participants of our study on the first day of classes how to use the mouse to click on the Start button and explaining to them what the Start menu was and what they could find there. In every subsequent training session, we would review this procedure and in fact even quiz the participants on the names of the icon and menu and when they were to be used. As an example, a popular quiz question was to ask participants at the beginning of class how to access the Internet from the desktop screen; by the end of the study, most participants would yell out in unison, "Go down to the bottom left and click on the Start button! And then click where it says 'Internet' in the Start menu!"

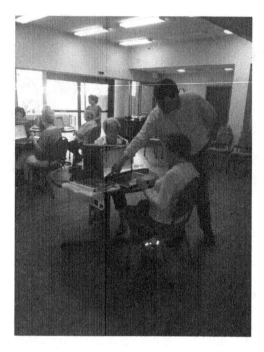

Figure 9.3 Instructor showing a study participant where the Start button is located on a laptop running the Windows Vista operating system.

This is how we progressed in each new CCRC we went to and conducted training sessions. And, because the Windows Vista operating system was unchanged, still popular, and still widely used in the beginning years of our study, we never encountered a major issue that led us to make major modifications to our training sessions or to our training manual in the middle of an 8-week training.

This changed, however, with the introduction of Windows 8. The Windows 8 operating system was released to the general public in 2012 and featured a completely new organizational and visual style compared to earlier Microsoft products. The Windows 8 operating system, rather than just updating the look and feel of previous Windows systems, instead opted to mirror the operating systems becoming popular on mobile and tablet technologies (in these systems, because there is no mouse or keyboard, programs are clustered together in different folders and packages usually located somewhere on the home screen of the device). A major change between Vista and Windows 8 was the elimination of the Start button that, in Vista, was always located at the bottom-left corner of the computer screen. Without a Start button, there was no Start menu, and to the uninitiated it was somewhat confusing as to where to locate a needed computer program.

This posed a problem for our ICT trainings in 2013. At one particular location, a resident purchased her own laptop computer for personal use and wanted assistance with learning to use it. Without seeing the laptop, our training staff initially assured her that we would be more than happy with assisting her during our office hours sessions and that all she needed to do was to bring the laptop with her to the session. Anytime a resident had a personal computer he or she wished to learn about, we would ask him or her to bring it to office hours rather than to class. When she arrived at the office hours session and opened her laptop, the first question out of her mouth was, "Well...where's the Start button?" As it turned out, her new laptop was running the Windows 8 operating system, and we had to tell her, "There is no Start button."

Things were further complicated in that the visual look of the Windows 8 operating system was completely different from that of Windows Vista, and the participant had a lot of trouble navigating without becoming confused (much of what she learned in class, such as where to find certain things on a screen, was no longer applicable). The fact that our training manual did not provide any instructions on using Windows 8 added to the complications, as the participant had nothing to take home with her to practice. Unfortunately, many new devices, software programs, and applications do not come with written documentation to help individuals, particularly older adults and less tech-savvy people, effectively learn to use them. Luckily for us, the participant was very understanding—she was aware that her new computer was truly *new* and that our training program was not designed to teach this new technology. Despite this, we asked her to keep coming to office hours sessions so that we could continue to assist her (and learn the intricacies of Windows 8 ourselves), and by the end of the study, she was able to accomplish many of the tasks we taught in the formal class sessions.

9.5.2   The move to mobile-friendly interfaces

The somewhat drastic change in look, feel, and navigability between Windows Vista and Windows 8 posed a significant issue for our training sessions, but changing interfaces are something that should be readily anticipated and planned for. It is up to the trainers to be well-versed in a variety of technologies and their latest versions in order to prevent instances like this, and having an updated training manual that accommodates these interfaces can go a long way in helping residents successfully learn and master the technology without becoming overwhelmed or confused.

The question thus arises: In what direction will future interfaces go? What should technology trainers prepare for? What will the typical interface be 1, 5, or 10 years from now?

The general trend we have seen in recent years has been the move from a more traditional, desktop-computer-based interface (complete with a mouse, keyboard, and—yes—a Start button!) to a mobile-friendly interface. By "mobile-friendly," we refer to an interface that is easily used and navigable on a mobile technology, such as a smartphone or a tablet computer. Examples of popular mobile technologies include the iPhone (a smartphone) and iPad (a tablet).

The biggest difference between a mobile interface and a more traditional desktop computer interface is that the mobile interface is specifically designed to not require the use of an external keyboard or a mouse, even though it is possible to purchase a keyboard and mouse to plug into mobile devices. Rather, the screens of these devices are actually touchscreens—the user may use his or her fingers or a stylus to navigate to different folders and different pages by touching certain icons or swiping his or her fingers across the screen. Mobile interfaces, because of this, tend to have a different organizational structure with regard to their programs (as mentioned earlier), such as having programs listed and accessible on the home page rather than having to access them through the use of a Start button or Start menu.

Mobile interfaces are becoming increasingly prevalent as mobile technologies become more and more popular. These interfaces also provide a unique and exciting avenue through which to teach older adults how to use Internet-connected devices. An example is a CCRC resident who has tremors and therefore has difficulty using a mouse who finds the touch-screen capabilities of a tablet to be easier to use. There are some trade-offs, however; as an example, in a study that examined older adults' use of iPads, Jayroe and Wolfram (2012) reported that new users had difficulty using the built-in, touchscreen keyboard compared to an external keyboard. However, research by Tsai and colleagues (Tsai et al., 2015) found that tablets were easier for older adults to learn to use than were traditional computers. Although no ICT will be perfect, tablets appear to offer advantages over other types of ICTs for older adults. See the Recommended Readings section at the end of this chapter for other research on tablet usage among older adults.

9.6   Robotics and telepresence

There is an episode from the popular CBS drama *The Good Wife*, a show about cases and internal conflicts of a Chicago-based law firm, in which a firm employee works with her colleagues through the use of a telepresence robot. The robot itself was essentially a tablet computer mounted on a pole on a small moving cart; the tablet allowed for the user to videoconference (i.e., the user could receive and transmit both audio and visual data) with the other employees of the firm, and the user could also remotely control the cart, allowing the user to move the tablet from room to room and follow the firm employees. Although the robot was played for laughs in the episode (with the robot constantly running into things or being shut out of meetings due to the user's inability to handle it properly), it provides an illustration of the potential of robotics and telepresence in everyday life.

The term "telepresence" refers to the ability of individuals to appear and act as if they were present in a certain location without actually being there. A popular form of telepresence that was discussed earlier in this chapter is achieved through videoconferencing, wherein an individual may transmit audio and visual data to another location. Whether through Skype, FaceTime, or another videoconferencing application, a user is not only able to hear the person he or she is talking to but can also see him or her. The user may not be in the room with the person he or she is talking to, but it *feels like* he or she is in the same room.

Technology developers in recent years have taken telepresence a step further by incorporating robotics. A telepresence robot allows for the user not only to transmit audio and visual data but also to move the robot around—in this way, the user can gather more information on a particular setting (e.g., survey the room of the person the user is communicating with) and communicate with more flexibility (e.g., moving the robot around to talk with different people in different locations). The different potential uses of telepresence robotics within health and healthcare are numerous, particularly for CCRC populations. Examples include, but are not limited to, the following:

- Having friends and family of a CCRC resident use a telepresence robot to visit and communicate with the resident remotely, which may be advantageous for individuals who live far away from their loved ones
- Having a CCRC resident use a telepresence robot to remotely "travel" outside of the CCRC, including attending classes at a local community center or going to a local church service
- Use of a telepresence robot for individuals who are not mobile to participate in CCRC activities within the community, whether it be bingo, dances, or other activities
- Having doctors and other healthcare professionals use telepresence robots to interact with CCRC patients when an in-person visit is inconvenient or impossible

9.7   The Internet of things

In addition to the telepresence, telepresence robots, and virtual healthcare opportunities that exist and are continually being improved upon in today's society, another important consideration regarding ICTs has to do with what is known as the Internet of things (IoT). The IoT refers to the multitude of devices and applications that are becoming increasingly pervasive in our society and how these things can work or be connected together. Companies are developing engineering and computing interfaces to help different Internet-enabled devices and applications "talk" to one another. Many can be implemented via mobile phones and tablet computers.

The IoT has significant potential for CCRCs and older adults more generally. For older adults to be as independent as possible, they may need assistance with various activities. For instance, they may move slower or have other mobility problems, which might make answering their door more difficult. Having their door fitted with a camera that shows the person at the door, as well as providing a means to unlock the door remotely, could help older adults with mobility problems. Other examples include an IoT-connected system to control temperature, lights, on and off switches, and so forth in homes. Others give medication reminders, detect changes in gait, sense movement in homes, monitor sleep and breathing, detect falls, detect onset of symptoms of particular diseases, and include emergency communication and contacts. They may connect sensors, doorbells, lighting controls, and so forth through a combination of wearable devices and smart home devices. Still others may involve remote monitoring of people and places. Inexpensive video monitoring systems allow caregivers to monitor the behavior and movement of individuals.

These tools can help older adults be more cognizant of their own health, have better control over their environment, and make better decisions about appropriate activities. They can also alert caregivers and CCRC staff of behaviors that indicate worsening health status, falls, accidents, wandering, and so forth. Although offering a range of potential benefits for residents and their caregivers, as well as CCRCs, privacy and security concerns may be an issue with older adults. Any CCRC or caregiver attempting to implement an IoT tool will need to discuss privacy and security concerns with the older adults.

For those with access to IoT products, there is potential to see benefits for residents, caregivers, and CCRC communities. With the increase in IoT-enabled products, we anticipate that the connection among products and devices will only continue to grow in the coming years.

9.8   Conclusion

Technology is evolving rapidly, with new services, devices, and applications constantly being introduced, and it can become overwhelming to try to keep up with it all. Having said that, it is important for CCRC staff and administrators to remain vigilant and educated regarding new technologies; doing so not only prevents services provided at the CCRC from going out of date but also ensures that residents have knowledge and access to devices and applications that can improve their quality of life and help maintain or even improve their health. The discussions in this chapter focused specifically on trends and technologies that may be of importance to residents; for an overview of technologies that may be applicable for trainers and researchers to investigate and possibly use in a CCRC setting, see the Recommended Readings section.

Recommended readings

Tablet usage among older adults

Tsai, H. S., Shillair, R., and Cotten, S. R. In press. Social support and "playing around": An examination of how older adults acquire digital literacy with tablet computers. *Journal of Applied Gerontology.* doi: 10.1177/0733464815609440.

Tsai, H. S., Shillair, R., Cotten, S. R., Winstead, V., and Yost, E. 2015. Getting grandma online: Are tablets the answer for increasing digital inclusion for older adults in the U.S.? *Educational Gerontology, 41,* 695–709.

Technologies applicable for researchers and trainers to use in a CCRC setting

Berkowsky, R. W. and Czaja, S. J. 2015. The use of technology in behavioral intervention research: Advantages and challenges. In L. N. Gitlin and S. J. Czaja (Eds), *Behavioral intervention research: designing, evaluating, and implementing* (pp. 119–136). New York: Springer.

Charness, N., Demiris, G., and Krupinski, E. 2011. *Designing telehealth for an aging population: a human factors perspective.* Boca Raton, Florida: CRC Press.

Czaja, S. J., Loewenstein, D., Schulz, R., Nair, S. N., and Perdomo, D. 2013. A videophone psychosocial intervention for dementia caregivers. *The American Journal of Geriatric Psychiatry, 21*(11), 1071–1081. doi: 10.1016/j.jagp.2013.02.019.

Magg, S. 2012. *CCRCs without walls: Care models of the future.* Retrieved from https://www.healthlawyers.org/Events/Programs/Materials/Documents/LTC12/papers/EE_maag.pdf

Mitzner, T. L., Chen, T. L., Kemp, C. C., and Rogers, W. A. 2014. Identifying the potential for robotics to assist older adults in different living environments. *International Journal of Social Robotics, 6*(2), 213–227.

World Health Organization. 2010. *Telemedicine: Opportunities and developments in member states.* Retrieved from http://www.who.int/goe/publications/goe_telemedicine_2010.pdf

chapter ten

Conclusions and final thoughts

10.1 Thoughts on implementing training programs for older adults

There are many people who would have you believe that older adults cannot or are not willing to learn to use ICTs. We reject this assertion. We have spent many years working with older adults, helping them overcome the digital divide. Older adults can and will cross the digital divide if they see the benefits and relevance of using ICTs in their lives, and they have adequate training to help them learn to use ICTs. They want to learn to use ICTs! The overarching goal of this book is to ultimately help older adults cross the digital divide to become engaged and proficient users of ICTs. We focus on older adults in CCRCs as we spent more than 5 years working in these communities to train residents to become proficient computer and Internet users, but the information is useful to any group preparing a training program for older adults.

Not all of the older adults who were part of our training became proficient users, but the opportunity to learn about computer and technology use was meaningful to them as well. It helped them to know that they were connected to the rest of the world because of the knowledge acquired through training. Not only did it prove to them that they could learn a new skill, but it also gave them the vocabulary necessary to converse in a meaningful way as a citizen of the technologically advanced twenty-first century. Even if they did not maintain their computer skills from the courses, there was still value in the training.

The purpose of this book is to provide a guide for others who wish to implement training programs in CCRCs. We wanted to tailor the material to help owners, administrators, and managers of CCRCs to think about the full range of considerations needed when trying to decide whether and how to train older adults to use ICTs. We believe that sharing our experiences in what worked and what did not work could be immensely helpful to those involved in formal or informal training sessions with older adults, particularly residents in CCRCs. We wanted this information to also be useful for technology designers who strive to develop and implement new gadgets, devices, and applications for older adults as well as for those who are nearing older age. We wanted these same individuals to understand the potential benefits to residents that technology use could offer.

In addition, the material presented here should be useful to researchers and policy makers who recognize the value of large-scale technology interventions and to those who work with older adults to examine factors that can help older adults to age successfully. Although it was daunting to write a book targeted at all these audiences, we think we have provided a useful resource that members of these groups will use to advance the successful aging and quality of life of older adults. In essence, this book serves as a case study to illuminate all of the issues that need to be considered to be successful in reaping the benefits of technology trainings and interventions in CCRCs.

Early chapters in this book discussed the demographic explosion in the older adult segment of the population in the United States and across the world, why and how technology use can be beneficial for older adults, and current trends in ICT use among older adults. Given the dramatic increase in the number of people turning 65 and older each day in recent years, as well as the projected increase in the number of people entering old age in the coming years, mechanisms are needed to help older adults maintain their independence and quality of life as they age. Isolation, loneliness, and depression increase among older adults, in addition to commonly expected declines in physical and cognitive health. Using ICTs may be one way to help older adults negate the negative effects of aging and to maintain their quality of life as they age. Through the use of ICTs, individuals can stay connected to geographically close and distant social ties, find information to help them make important life decisions, overcome social and spatial barriers, and stay connected to our larger information-based society.

In Chapter 2, we discussed the characteristics of CCRC communities, noting the range of services provided by these communities for residents. Individuals are waiting longer to move into CCRCs, as many people strive to age in place. By the time people move into CCRCs, and particularly into assisted living communities, many of them are frailer than were individuals 15 years ago or thereabouts who were moving into these communities. This presents challenges for those who seek to train older adults in CCRCs to use ICTs. However, this also makes the skills all the more relevant to overcoming issues of frailty.

Chapters 3 and 4 detailed our prototype study in which we trained older adults in assisted and independent living communities to use ICTs. These chapters also described best practices for and complexities of implementing technology training programs in CCRCs. We noted important factors to consider when deciding whether to conduct an ICT training in CCRCs, paying particular attention to how to engage residents, the staging of the training, and environmental factors. CCRCs are complex organizations. Having staff and administrators who see the value in ICT training is a key factor that can help predict success in the recruitment and retention of residents to training programs and the overall success of training programs. Adhering to these suggestions will help ensure that ICT training programs will fit the needs of the residents.

Although this training is a significant investment in terms of time, energy, and money, the resulting gains are considerable. Chapter 5 details the benefits to users. Findings from our longitudinal study showcase how simply identifying as a user can impact the quality of life and other mental health outcomes for a given older adult. It further discusses how the use of ICTs can change attitudes toward use and impact self-efficacy. Chapter 6 detailed best practices for recruitment and retention in ICT training programs.

For CCRC administrators and staff members who are interested in having their residents gain ICT use and skills, they need to decide whether to do training via someone internal to the CCRC or contract it to an outside organization. There are pros and cons with each of these approaches. Chapter 7 detailed factors to consider when deciding whether to do the training internally or through an external organization, as well as provided suggestions for how to find external organizations who could help CCRCs with training initiatives. The key, regardless of whether the trainers are internal or external, is to have trainers who are effective communicators and who relate well to older adults. The trainers also need to have an understanding of the barriers to learning and usage faced by many CCRC residents. Even good communicators will be unsuccessful in providing technology training if they fail to understand some of the unique issues that older learners must overcome in learning how to use technology.

Although it may seem obvious, the issue of Internet access is important in thinking about ICT training in CCRCs, a topic that was also covered in Chapter 7. Several of the communities where we did our training had Internet access, but we often needed to extend the range and make it wireless to effectively use it in our training sessions. In order for CCRC residents to maintain ICT use and skills they have developed through training, they need to have access to the Internet and to devices.

In Chapter 8, we discussed how needs and ICT use are changing for older adults. This includes the cost, method of access, support, and system interface. Financial challenges may make it impossible for residents to pay for their access, so it is important that CCRCs provide access to Wi-Fi throughout the community if possible, but at least in the common areas that offer comfortable and private places for residents to sit and use their devices. In our training, we provided desktop computers to CCRCs that the residents could use during and after our training sessions ended. If residents are not able to continue use, the skills they have acquired will deteriorate quickly.

In a similar vein, it may be necessary for CCRCs to maintain some type of ICT assistance within the community when residents have problems after the training programs have ended. Our experiences indicate that this often occurs, particularly when software updates occur or when new devices are purchased. We found anecdotally that the older adults were more likely to continue using ICTs if they had someone in their CCRC or a family member who could troubleshoot for them or provide continued ICT education, even informally.

In Chapter 9, we tried to think proactively about the future of technology and issues that will affect training older adults in CCRCs to use ICTs. We noted some of the anticipated issues, but technology development moves at such a fast pace it is likely that there will be many more developments that can benefit older adults, as well as significantly affect training programs, within a short period of time. CCRCs, as well as those helping older adults to cross the digital divide, want to stay abreast of the latest technology enhancements that can make life easier for older adults. CCRCs and trainers also want to stay informed and familiar with problems that may arise from these enhancements, such as updating training protocols when a new interface is introduced.

Having Wi-Fi access throughout CCRCs, ensuring privacy concerns are addressed, and providing materials via an intranet may help encourage residents to use ICTs in CCRCs. This is not only beneficial to residents but can also be beneficial to the administration and staff because of time and effort saved in the communication and dissemination of information throughout individual CCRCs. In addition, newer software and hardware developments are making it increasingly easier for older adults to learn to use ICTs. Voice recognition, touch-based interfaces, and virtual reality are three technology developments that we anticipate being particularly applicable to older adults in the future. Touch-based interfaces are already becoming increasingly used with tablet use among older adults. Although this interface does not resolve all issues for older adults in using ICTs, it can help many older adults overcome barriers to using ICTs associated with the use of a keyboard, mouse, and clicking. Mobile devices are also increasingly being used by older adults. The ease of use and portability makes mobile devices especially attractive options for older adults, but there is an added design challenge of the smaller size reducing the display space.

The potential for mobile health, or mHealth, applications through mobile devices is strong. Similarly, the Internet of things (IOT) has the potential to improve the quality of life for many older adults by linking together multiple devices to enable older adults to function more effectively in their homes and larger environments. In addition, recent studies have found evidence that novel and diverse activities may be useful in mitigating the effects of cognitive decline in older adults. What better resource for novelty and diversity than the Internet? When older adults are equipped with the tools for technology use, the benefits to them, cognitively and socially, and to their health are numerous.

Many companies do not currently focus on older adults when designing new devices. We encourage them to begin to focus on this vastly expanding demographic group. Each new generation of older adults will face many of the same challenges we observed in the older adults in our training. Lack of previous computer use will be less of an issue, but keeping up with new technology will always be a challenge for those in their later years. We encourage these companies to partner together to provide resources that will enable older adults to maintain a high quality of life, especially through technology that is accessible and usable for older adults, rather than each trying to develop the latest device or app that will revolutionize the way older adults use ICTs.

10.2   Further considerations and reflections

We are often asked: If we could do this all over, what would we change? This text details the best practices in teaching older adults in using ICTs, training design, and the lessons we learned during the process. We contend that our ICT training sessions were successful in educating older adults in CCRCs to use technology and in promoting increased quality of life. However, no training we conducted was perfect. Unfortunately, there is no single method of approaching and teaching CCRC residents when it comes to ICTs. Each community or group responsible for ICT training needs to tailor its classes to its own needs as well as the needs and preferences of the CCRC residents. These will change between CCRCs and will change over time as the makeup of the community changes or new technologies are introduced into the public sphere; however, the best practices outlined in this book will always be good guideposts.

Regarding what we would have changed: for our purposes, we would have preferred more time with study participants. Although participants had the option to call us for technical support for a period of time, after the training sessions were complete in the CCRC, in-person learning and practice seems to work better for this particular population. Had there been additional time and resources, once-a-month office hours or an in-person technical support system for an additional year or so would have been excellent. We discuss in this book how some CCRCs mitigated the problems associated with our decreased involvement by creating their own computer clubs so that residents could provide technical support to one another; however, although these groups promoted a sense of community and helped with minor troubleshooting issues, having our trainers be more available after the intervention would have promoted increased ICT use as well as possibly more advanced use.

The ICT marketplace is vast and growing, and technology changes quickly. During our study, we saw multiple new technology fads, designs, and updates to our major operating systems. Having separate groups or classes that covered different devices or operating systems (e.g., Apple devices, Android devices, PC computers) or having supplemental training materials (e.g., multiple training manuals covering different operating systems) could help give participants the information they would need to successfully get online regardless of the device they end up using. This requires additional work from trainers, as new classes need to be developed and additional supplemental materials need to be developed, but it would help alleviate issues that arise from switching devices (we highlighted one such issue in Chapter 9 wherein a study participant had trouble with using a device running the Windows 8 operating system after being trained to use a device running Windows Vista).

Not only does technology change quickly, but the CCRC resident also changes quickly. Having ways to continually adapt the technology to meet the needs of the CCRC population would be tremendously useful. Although an illness might cause a resident to not want to use the computer, perhaps there is a way to address this gap in use, such as bringing the office hours to the resident (i.e., having training sessions conducted in his or her room).

No training will ever be perfect. There will always be unforeseen issues and complications. Part of carrying out a successful training mandates that the trainers be cognizant of potential problems and be willing to "go with the flow" of the students at some point. As an example, residents at a particular CCRC may not be interested in learning about websites such as Hulu or YouTube; in this instance, it is better to keep them interested and reinforce what they want to learn rather than cover all-new material.

In conclusion, we hope readers of this book find the material presented useful as they work with older adults, through training them to use ICTs, designing new technologies to benefit older adults, or studying how to enhance successful aging among older adults. Finally, we hope that owners, administrators, and staff of CCRCs will find this book informative as they think about the future of older adults in their communities. Here's to a future with many more older adults using ICTs to help them stay connected with their social ties, find information to make important life decisions, and stay engaged in the larger social world of which they are a part.

Bibliography

AARP. 2015. *About continuing care retirement communities.* Retrieved from http://www.aarp.org/relationships/caregiving-resource-center/info-09-2010/ho_continuing_care_retirement_communities.html

American Telemedicine Association. 2015. *Research outcomes: Telemedicine's impact on healthcare cost and quality.* Retrieved from http://www.americantelemed.org/docs/default-source/policy/examples-of-research-outcomes—telemedicine's-impact-on-healthcare-cost-and-quality.pdf

Assisted Living Federation of America. 2013. *What is assisted living?* Retrieved June 15, 2013, from http://www.alfa.org/alfa/Assisted_Living_Information.asp

Bandura, A. 1982. Self-efficacy mechanism in human agency. *American Psychologist, 37,* 122–147.

Berkowsky, R. W. 2012. Internet use, social integration, and psychological well-being in older adults (Master's thesis). The University of Alabama, Birmingham.

Berkowsky, R. W. 2014. Internet use and mental health/well-being in old age: Exploring the roles of social integration and social support (Doctoral dissertation). The University of Alabama, Birmingham.

Berkowsky, R. W., Cotten, S. R., Yost, E. A., and Winstead, V. P. 2013. Attitudes towards and limitations to ICT use in assisted and independent living communities: Findings from a specially-designed technological intervention. *Educational Gerontology, 39,* 797–811.

Berkowsky, R. W. and Czaja, S. J. 2015. The use of technology in behavioral intervention research: Advantages and challenges. In L. N. Gitlin and S. J. Czaja (Eds.), *Behavioral intervention research: Designing, evaluating, and implementing* (pp. 119–136). New York: Springer.

Bhamra, S., Tinker, A., Mein, G., Ashcroft, R., and Askham, J. 2008. The retention of older people in longitudinal studies: A review of the literature. *Quality in Ageing, 9,* 27–35.

Boulton-Lewis, G. M. 2010. Education and learning for the elderly: Why, how, what. *Educational Gerontology, 36,* 213–228.

Caffrey, C., Sengupta, M., Park-Lee, E., Moss, A., Rosenoff, E., and Harris-Kojetin, L. 2012. *Residents living in residential care facilities: United States, 2010* (NCHS Data Brief 91). Hyattsville, Maryland: National Center for Health Statistics.

Center for Connected Health Policy. n.d. *What is teleheath?* Retrieved from http://cchpca.org/what-is-telehealth

Chaffin, A. J. and Harlow, S. D. 2005. Cognitive learning applied to older adult learners and technology. *Educational Gerontology, 31,* 301–329.

Charness, N., Demiris, G., and Krupinski, E. 2011. *Designing telehealth for an aging population: A human factors perspective.* Boca Raton, Florida: CRC Press.

Cody, M. J., Dunn, D., Hoppin, S., and Wendt, P. 1999. Silver surfers: Training and evaluating internet use among older adult learners. *Communication Education, 48,* 269–286.

Cotten, S. R., Anderson, W. A., and McCullough, B. M. 2013. Impact of Internet use on loneliness and contact with others among older adults: Cross-sectional analysis. *Journal of Medical Internet Research, 15*(2), e39. doi: 10.2196/jmir.2306.

Cutchin, M. P., Owen, S. V., and Chang, P.-F. J. 2003. Becoming "at home" in assisted living residences: Exploring place integration processes. *Journals of Gerontology: Social Sciences, 58B*(4), S234–S243.

Czaja, S. J., Loewenstein, D., Schulz, R., Nair, S. N., and Perdomo, D. 2013. A videophone psychosocial intervention for dementia caregivers. *The American Journal of Geriatric Psychiatry, 21*(11), 1071–1081. doi: 10.1016/j.jagp.2013.02.019.

Czaja, S. J. and Sharit, J. 2013. *Designing training and instructional programs for older adults.* Boca Raton, Florida: CRC Press.

Davies, S. L., Goodman, C., Manthorpe, J., Smith, A., Carrick, N., and Iliffe, S. 2014. Enabling research in care homes: An evaluation of a national network of research ready care homes. *BMC Medical Research Methodology, 14,* 47. doi: 10.1186/1471-2288-14-47.

Davison, E. and Cotten, S. R. 2003. Connection discrepancies: Unmasking further layers of the digital divide. *First Monday, 8*(3). http://dx.doi.org/10.5210/fm.v8i3.1039

Davison, E. and Cotten, S. R. 2010. Connection disparities: The importance of broadband connections in understanding today's digital divide. In E. Ferro, Y. Dwivedi, J. Gil-Garcia, and M. D. Williams (Eds.), *Overcoming digital divides: Constructing an equitable and competitive information society* (pp. 346–358). Hershey, Pennsylvania: IGI Global.

Dobriansky, P. J., Suzman, R. M., and Hodes, R. J. 2007. *Why population aging matters: A global perspective* (Publication 07-6134). Washington, DC: National Institute on Aging, National Institutes of Health, US Department of Health and Human Services, US Department of State.

Duay, D. L. and Bryan, V. C. 2008. Learning in later life: What seniors want in a learning experience. *Educational Gerontology, 34,* 1070–1086.

Dupuis-Blanchard, S., Neufeld, A., and Strang, V. R. 2009. The significance of social engagement in relocated older adults. *Qualitative Health Research, 19*(9), 1186–1195.

Eckert, J. K., Carder, P. C., Morgan, L. A., Frankowski, A. C., and Roth, E. G. 2009. *Inside assisted living: The search for home.* Baltimore, Maryland: Johns Hopkins University Press.

Fisk, A. D., Rogers, W. A., Charness, N., Czaja, S. J., and Sharit, J. 2009. *Designing for older adults: Principles and creative human factors approaches* (2nd ed.). Boca Raton, Florida: CRC Press.

Green, L. 2010. *The internet: An introduction to new media.* New York: Berg.

Hays, J. C. 2002. Living arrangements and health status in later life: A review of recent literature. *Public Health Nursing, 19*(2), 136–151.

Heisler, E., Evans, G. W., and Moen, P. 2003. Health and social outcomes of moving to a continuing care retirement community. *Journal of Housing for the Elderly, 18*(1), 5–23.

Heo, J., Chun, S., Lee, S., Lee, K. H., and Kim, J. 2015. Internet use and well-being in older adults. *Cyberpsychology, Behavior, and Social Networking, 18*(5), 268–272. doi:10.1089/cyber.2014.0549.

Horrigan, J. B. and Duggan, M. 2015. *Home broadband 2015.* Pew Research Center. Retrieved from http://www.pewinternet.org/files/2015/12/Broadband-adoption-full.pdf

Jayroe, T. J. and Wolfram, D. 2012. Internet searching, tablet technology and older adults. *Proceedings of the American Society for Information Science and Technology, 49*, 1–3.

Kane, R. A. 2001. Long-term care and a good quality of life: Bringing them closer together. *The Gerontologist, 41*, 293–304.

Kane, R. A. and Wilson, K. B. 1993. *Assisted living in the United States: A new paradigm for residential care for frail older persons?* Washington, DC: American Association of Retired Persons.

Karavidas, M., Lim, N. K., and Katsikas, S. L. 2005. The effects of computers on older adult users. *Computers in Human Behavior, 21*(5), 697–711.

LeadingAge Ziegler 150. 2014. Retrieved from https://www.leadingage.org/uploadedFiles/Content/Members/Member_Services/LZ_100/LZ150-2014.pdf

Magg, S. 2012. *CCRCs without walls: Care models of the future.* Retrieved from https://www.healthlawyers.org/Events/Programs/Materials/Documents/LTC12/papers/EE_maag.pdf

Marsden, J. 2005. *Humanistic designs of assisted living.* Baltimore, Maryland: Johns Hopkins University Press.

McHenry, J. C., Insel, K. C., Einstein, G. O., Vidrine, A. N., Koerner, K. M., and Morrow, D. G. 2015. Recruitment of older adults: Success may be in the details. *The Gerontologist, 55*(5), 845–853.

McNeely, E. A. and Clements, S. D. 1994. Recruitment and retention of the older adults into research studies. *Journal of Neuroscience Nursing, 26*, 57–61.

Millward, P. 2003. The "grey digital divide": Perception, exclusion and barriers of access to the internet for older people. *First Monday, 8*(7). doi: 10.5210/fm.v8i7.1066.

Mitzner, T. L., Chen, T. L., Kemp, C. C., and Rogers, W. A. 2014. Identifying the potential for robotics to assist older adults in different living environments. *International Journal of Social Robotics, 6*(2), 213–227.

Namazi, K. H. and McClintic, M. 2003. Computer use among elderly persons in long-term care facilities. *Educational Gerontology, 29*(6), 535–550.

Ortmann, J., Velkoff, V., and Hogan, H. 2014. *An Aging Nation: The Older Population in the United States* (Current Population Reports P25-1140). Washington, DC: US Census Bureau.

Pak, R. and McLaughlin, A. C. 2010. *Designing displays for older adults.* Boca Raton, Florida: CRC Press.

Perrin, A. and Duggan, M. 2015. *Americans' Internet access: 2000–2015.* Washington, DC: Pew Research Center. Retrieved from http://www.pewinternet.org/2015/06/26/americans-internet-access-2000-2015/

Purdie, N. and Boulton-Lewis, G. 2003. The learning needs of older adults. *Educational Gerontology, 29*(2), 129–149.

Reich, W. T. 1978. Ethical issues related to research involving elderly subjects. *The Gerontologist, 18*(4), 326–337.

Richardson, M., Zorn, T. E., Jr., and Weaver, K. 2002. *Seniors' perspectives on the barriers, benefits and negatives consequences of learning and using computers.* Hamilton, New Zealand: Department of Management Communication, Waikato Management School.

Rogers, W. A., Campbell, R. H., and Pak, R. 2001. A systems approach for training older adults to use technology. In N. Charness, D. C. Parks, and B. A. Sabel (Eds.), *Communication, technology and aging—Opportunities and challenges for the future* (pp. 187–208). New York: Springer.

Rogers, W. A., and Fisk, A. D. 2010. Toward a psychological science of advanced technology design for older adults. *The Journals of Gerontology Series B: Psychological Sciences and Social Sciences, 65B*(6), 645–653. http://doi.org/10.1093/geronb/gbq065

Romero, N., Sturm, J., Bekker, T., de Valk, L., and Kruitwagen, S. 2010. Playful persuasion to support older adults' social and physical activities. *Interacting with Computers, 22*, 485–495.

Rosenthal, R. L. 2008. Older computer-literate women: Their motivations, obstacles, and paths to success. *Educational Gerontology, 34*(7), 610–626.

Ryff, C. D. 1989. Happiness is everything, or is it? Explorations on the meaning of psychological well-being. *Journal of Personality and Social Psychology, 57*(6), 1069–1081.

Shearer, N., Fleury, J., and Belyea, M. 2008. An innovative approach to recruiting homebound older adults. *Journal of the American Geriatrics Society, 56*(12), 2340–2348.

Sixsmith, A. and Gutman, G. 2013. *Technologies for active aging.* New York: Springer.

Sloane, P. D., Zimmerman, S., and Walsh, J. F. 2001. The physical environment. In S. Zimmerman, P. D. Sloane, and J. K. Eckert (Eds.), *Assisted living: Needs, practices and policies in residential care for the elderly* (pp. 173–197). Baltimore, Maryland: Johns Hopkins University Press.

Smith, A. 2014. *Older adults and technology use.* Washington, DC: Pew Research Center. Retrieved from http://www.pewinternet.org/2014/04/03/older-adults-and-technology-use/

Stevens, B. 2003. How seniors learn. *Issue Brief: Center for Medicare Education, 4*(9), 1–8.

Stula, S. 2012. Living in old age in Europe—Current developments and challenges. Working Paper No. 7 of the Observatory for Sociopolitical Developments in Europe. Berlin, Germany: German Association for Public and Private Welfare (DV). Retrieved from http://www.sociopolitical-observatory.eu/uploads/tx_aebgppublications/AP_7_EN.pdf

Suzman, R. and Beard, J. 2011. *Global health and aging* (NIH Publication No. 11-7737). Washington, DC: National Institutes of Health and World Health Organization.

Swezey, R. W. and Llaneras, R. E. 1997. Models in training and instruction. In G. Salvendy (Ed.), *Handbook of human factors and ergonomics* (2nd ed., pp. 514–577). New York: Wiley.

Tsai, H. S., Shillair, R., and Cotten, S. R. In press. Social support and "playing around": An examination of how older adults acquire digital literacy with tablet computers. *Journal of Applied Gerontology*. doi: 10.1177/0733464815609440.

Tsai, H. S., Shillair, R., Cotten, S. R., Winstead, V., and Yost, E. 2015. Getting grandma online: Are tablets the answer for increasing digital inclusion for older adults in the U.S.? *Educational Gerontology, 41*, 695–709.

United Nations, Department of Economic and Social Affairs, Population Division 2013. *World population ageing 2013* (ST/ESA/SER.A/348). Retrieved from http://www.un.org/en/development/desa/population/publications/pdf/ageing/WorldPopulationAgeing2013.pdf

Wagner, N., Hassanein, K., and Head, M. 2010. Computer use by older adults: A multi-disciplinary review. *Computers in Human Behavior, 26*, 870–882.

Waldron, V. R., Gitelson, R., and Kelley, D. L. 2005. Gender differences in social adaptation to a retirement community: Longitudinal changes and the role of mediated communication. *Journal of Applied Gerontology, 24*(4), 283–298.

Wilson, K. B. 2007. Historical evolution of assisted living in the United States, 1979 to the present. *The Gerontologist, 47*(suppl 1), 8–22.

Winstead, V. and Anderson, W. A., Yost, E. A., Cotten, S. R., Warr, A., and Berkowsky, R. W. 2013. You can teach an old dog new tricks: A qualitative analysis of how residents of senior living communities may use the web to overcome spatial and social barriers. *Journal of Applied Gerontology, 32*(5), 540–560.

Wood, F., Prout, H., Bayer, A., Duncan, D., Nuttall, J., Hood, K., and Butler, C. C. 2013. Consent, including advanced consent, of older adults to research in care homes: A qualitative study of stakeholders' views in South Wales. *Trials, 14*, 247. doi: 10.1186/1745-6215-14-247.

Woodward, A. M., Freddolino, P. P., Wishart, D. J., Bakk, L., Kobayashi, R., Tupper, C., Panci, J., and Blaschke-Thompson, C. M. 2013. Outcomes from a peer tutor model for teaching technology to older adults. *Ageing and Society, 33*, 1315–1338.

World Health Organization. 2010. *Telemedicine: Opportunities and developments in member states*. Retrieved from http://www.who.int/goe/publications/goe_telemedicine_2010.pdf

Wrights, A. P., Fain, C. W., Miller, M. E., Rejeski, W. J., Williamson, J. D., and Marsh, A. P. 2015. Assessing physical and cognitive function of older adults in continuing care retirement communities: Who are we recruiting? *Contemporary Clinical Trials, 40*, 159–165. doi: 10.1016/j.cct.2014.12.003.

Xie, B. 2007. Information technology education for older adults as a continuing peer-learning process: A Chinese case study. *Educational Gerontology, 33*, 429–450.

Yamasaki, J. and Sharf, B. F. 2011. Opting out and fitting in: How residents make sense of assisted living and cope with community life. *Journal of Aging Studies, 23*, 13–21.

Zarem, J. E. 2010. *Today's continuing care retirement community (CCRC)*. LeadingAge and American Seniors Housing Association. Retrieved from https://www.leadingage.org/uploadedFiles/Content/Consumers/Paying_for_Aging_Services/CCRCcharacteristics_7_2011.pdf

Zheng, R. Z., Hill, R. D., and Gardner M. K. 2013. *Engaging older adults with modern technology: Internet use and information access needs*. Hershey, Pennsylvania: IGI Global.

Appendix

Sample ICT training curriculum for CCRC residents[a]

Week	Day	Topic	Objectives	Notes
Week 1	Day 1	Computer basics (I)	By the end of the session, residents will have a better understanding of: • Computer terminology • Basic components of the computer • How to turn a computer on • How to use a mouse • How to access the Start menu • How to open and close applications and windows • How to shut down a computer	Use an online mouse training program, such as www.mouseprogram.com, to familiarize residents with the basic use and functions of the mouse.
	Day 2	Computer basics (II)	By the end of the session, residents will have a better understanding of: • How to access programs from the Start menu • How to access folders from the Start menu • How to access and play games	Have residents play a computer game they may already be familiar with, such as solitaire.
Week 2	Day 1	Creating an email account	By the end of the session, residents will have a better understanding of: • How to get online • What email and Gmail are • How to navigate to Gmail • How to create a Gmail account	Residents should write down their Gmail username and password for future use; it is recommended the training staff should also have copies of Gmail credentials in case residents lose or forget their login information.

(Continued)

Sample ICT training curriculum for CCRC residents[a]

Week	Day	Topic	Objectives	Notes
	Day 2	The basics of using email	By the end of the session, residents will have a better understanding of: • How to log into/out of Gmail • How to read email • How to compose and send email	Have residents compose and send an email to a dummy account (e.g., an email account created by the trainers specifically for class).
Week 3	Day 1	Introduction to the Internet (I)	By the end of the session, residents will have a better understanding of: • What a search engine such as Google is • How to use a search engine to find information and websites • What a URL is • How to use the URL/address bar to navigate to a website	Possible topics to search for include recipes, news, and the weather. When teaching the residents how to use the address bar to navigate to a website, a site with a simple URL (e.g., cnn.com) is recommended.
	Day 2	Introduction to the Internet (II)	By the end of the session, residents will have a better understanding of: • What the different types of websites that can be found online are • What the most frequently used domains (e.g., .com, .edu, .gov, .org, .net) are	Provide examples of different types of sites and have the residents navigate to them using Google and the address bar to help review these skills.
Week 4	Day 1	Advanced email (I)	By the end of the session, residents will have a better understanding of: • How to forward email • How to open and save attachments	Trainers should email all residents a practice email with attachments to open and save, such as humorous pictures.

(*Continued*)

Sample ICT training curriculum for CCRC residents[a]

Week	Day	Topic	Objectives	Notes
	Day 2	Advanced email (II)	By the end of the session, residents will have a better understanding of: • How to compose email with attachments	Residents should practice attaching files using pictures saved on the computer (either sample pictures or the pictures downloaded from the previous class).
Week 5	Day 1	Social network websites	By the end of the session, residents will have a better understanding of: • What social networking is • Facebook • Twitter • Social network aspects of the AARP site	This session is presented in lecture format. If there is enough time at the end of the session and residents are interested in any of the sites, trainers may assist residents with creating accounts.
	Day 2	Practice day	This session addresses questions from residents and provides free time for practice.	During free time, residents may play games, use email, or go online.
Week 6	Day 1	Health information on the web	By the end of the session, residents will have a better understanding of: • How to look for health information • How to evaluate trustworthiness of a website • What some popular sources of health information are	The "Evaluating Health Information on the World Wide Web" guide developed by the SPRY Foundation (www.spry.org) can be used for reference by both the trainers and residents.
	Day 2	Practice day	This session addresses questions from residents and provides free time for practice.	During free time, residents may play games, use email, or go online.
Week 7	Day 1	Entertainment websites	By the end of the session, residents will have a better understanding of: • How to use Hulu to search for and watch television programs and films • How to use YouTube to search for and watch entertaining videos	To promote engagement, it is recommended that trainers expose residents to videos they may have interest in (e.g., old television programs such as *Bewitched*).

(Continued)

Sample ICT training curriculum for CCRC residents[a]

Week	Day	Topic	Objectives	Notes
	Day 2	Practice day	This session addresses questions from residents and provides free time for practice.	During free time, residents may play games, use email, or go online.
Week 8	Day 1	Final project (I)	This session incorporates a final project that reviews various skills covered over the previous weeks. After being given a topic, residents must: • Find a website that gives information on the provided topic • Copy the URL of the website • Open Gmail and compose an email, pasting the previously copied URL into the email • Send the email	In this session, the trainers review with the residents the step-by-step procedures needed to accomplish the final project. Everyone in the class does the project together at the same pace.
	Day 2	Final project (II)	On the last day of class, residents repeat the final project from the previous session.	In this session, residents are instructed to complete the project on their own. Trainers are made available in case residents have questions or if anyone has problems completing the project.

[a] The outlined curriculum was developed for an 8-week training course in the basics of using ICTs, specifically the basics of using a desktop or laptop computer and using the Internet, for CCRC residents. Residents met for training twice per week, with each session lasting approximately 90 minutes. Each class session began with a review of what participants had learned in the prior class; each class ended with a review of what participants had learned in that particular training session.

Index

A

Access, 143–144, 157–160
Activities of daily living (ADLs), 15, 19
Activity directors, 105–106
    in recruitment and retention, 120–121
Aging
    in place, 22, 36
    process, 25
Aging population demographics, 2
    China, 6
    global population pyramid, 4
    global trends, 2
    population pyramid for Japan, 5
    U.S. trends, 6–9
    world population and percentage, 3
AL, *see* Assisted living
ALCs, *see* Assisted living communities
Anticipated numbers, 127–129
Assisted living (AL), 112
Assisted living communities (ALCs), 11,
    18–20, 56
Assistive devices, 38–39, 47
Audio visual equipment (AV equipment), 44

B

Best practices, *see* Complexities and best
    practices for CCRC
Broadband, 157–160
    Internet access, 157
Building rapport, 115–116

C

Care community analogues abroad, 20–21
Caveats, 134–135

CCRCs, *see* Continuing care retirement
    communities
China, population in, 6
Chronic health issues, management of, 156
Class time, 116–119
Cloud-based systems, 144
Cognitive
    ability, 59–61
    barriers, 106, 115
    limitations, 126
    screener, 115
Community, 105
    meetings, 109
Complexities and best practices for
    CCRC; *see also* Continuing
    care retirement communities
    (CCRCs)
    cognitive ability, 59–61
    designing and presenting content, 67
    dexterity, 58–59
    enabling older adult to adapting
        rapidly changing technology,
        76–78
    engaging activity directors, 75–76
    engaging and motivating participants, 70
    ensuring equipment, 64–67
    expecting attrition, 78–79
    hearing ability, 58–59
    learner, 56
    to lecture, 68
    organizing environment, 61
    other considerations, 75
    physical health and mobility of older
        learners, 57–58
    physical layout of classroom, 61–63
    practices, 72–73
    promoting community, 73–75

Complexities and best practices for CCRC
        (*Continued*)
    scheduling, 63–64
    supportive teaching team, 71–72
    taking content home, 68–69
    technology instructors, 55–56
    training trainer, 70–71
    visual ability, 58–59
Computers, 150
    training, 110
Confidence, 89
Confidentiality, 152
Continual support, 144–145
Continuing care retirement communities
        (CCRCs), 1, 15, 55, 103, 108, 109,
        125, 131, 141–142, 151, 153
    access, 143–144
    aging population demographics, 2–8
    care community analogues abroad,
        20–21
    continual support, 144–145
    development of, 17
    ILCs *vs.* ALCs, 18–20
    interface, 141–143
    keep it simple, 144
    model, 15–17
    older adults and technology usage,
        26–30
    outsiders for continued use, 146–147
    population, fit with, 140
    recruiting at different care levels,
        112–113
    residential communities for older
        adults, 11–12
    statistics on ILCs and ALCs, 18
    stress of transition, 22–26
    technology training for older adults
        in, 1–2
    technology using older adults, 9–11
    value of technology for older adults, 9
"Continuing education" training, 143
Cost, 139
Cover entertainment websites, 67
Crisis, 22

D

Depression, 94–96
Designing training sessions, 130
Dexterity, 58–59
Dial-up connection, 157
Digital divide, 9, 64, 72, 84

E

Eagle Eye (film), 150
Education, 10
Elderspeak, 116
Email system, 153
Emergency response systems, 156
Emotional needs, 114
Entertainment websites, 50
Eschewing esoteric metaphors, 144
European Union (EU), care community
        analogues, 20
External contractor decisions,
        136–139

F

Facebook, 67
FaceTime, 146
Family council meetings, 109
Fee-for-service contract, 16
Fit with CCRC population, 140
Flyer, 109
Formal recruitment, 106
        sessions, 106–108

G

Gerontocomia, 17
Google, 83
Group training sessions, 129–130

H

Health
    declines, 126
    education, 154
    promotion applications, 156
Healthcare
    delivery, 154
    via teleconferencing, 154–155
    via videoconferencing, 154–155
Hearing ability, 58–59

I

IADLs, *see* Instrumental activities of daily
        living
ICTs, *see* Information and communication
        technologies
IL, *see* Independent living
ILCs, *see* Independent living communities

Incentives in recruitment and retention for
    research projects, 121–122
Independent living (IL), 112
Independent living communities (ILCs),
    11, 18–20, 56
Individual training sessions, 129–130
Informal recruitment sessions,
    109–110
Information and communication
    technologies (ICTs), 2, 84, 109,
    125, 153
Information repetition method, 60
Instrumental activities of daily living
    (IADLs), 19
Interface, 141–143, 160
    mobile-friendly interfaces, 163–164
    trouble with going from Windows
        Vista to Windows 8, 160–163
Internet, 9, 28, 67, 103
    Internet-connected system, 154
Internet of things (IoT), 165–166
Interpersonal characteristics, 132–134
Intranet, 151–154
IoT, *see* Internet of things

L

Life care contract, 16
Loneliness, 94–96

M

Matrix, The, 150
Medication adherence, 156
mHealt, 156
Mini Mental Status Examination (MMSE),
    115
Minority Report (film), 149
MMSE, *see* Mini Mental Status
    Examination
Mobile
    health applications, 155–157
    learning applications, 156
    mobile-friendly interfaces, 163–164
Mobility, 57
Modified contract, 16

N

National Institute on Aging (NIA), 35
Needs, retention, 114–115
Noncognitive factors, 58

O

Office hours, 119–120
Older adults, 103, 125, 146
    barriers to older adults in CCRC,
        28–29
    changing interfaces, 160–164
    developments in world of technology,
        149–151
    increased access and importance of
        broadband, 157–160
    Internet accessing, 28
    intranet, 151–154
    IoT, 165–166
    long-term care, 27
    robotics and telepresence,
        164–165
    technology usage, 26–27
    and technology usage, 26
    technology usage and connection to
        modern society, 29–30
    virtual healthcare, 154–157

P

Pamphlet, 109
Physical access, 143
Physical barriers, 106
Physical limitations, 126
Piggybacking, 106
Pilot testing, 142–143
Posttraining evaluations, 133–134
PreCrime, 149
Primary trainer, 134
Prototype study
    assessment, 51–52
    assistive devices, 38–39, 47
    find lots of room, 41–44
    gaining entrance, 34–35
    idea for, 33–34
    implementation, 47–49
    lessons learning, 52–53
    preparation, 36
    recruiting process, 40–41
    reducing distractions and frustrations,
        46–47
    reimaging, 38
    retention, 49–51
    scheduling and fitting into CCRC
        schedules, 44–46
    selecting context, 35–36
    staging intervention, 41

Prototype study (*Continued*)
    training and self-education, 36–37
    training manual table of contents, 37
Psychological well-being, 96–97

Q

Quality of life outcomes, 94
    case study, 98–99
    depression and loneliness, 94–96
    psychological well-being, 96–97
    spatial barriers, social barriers and
        connecting with others, 97
"Queen of activity directors", 120

R

Recruitment, 103
    activity director, 120–121
    at care levels of CCRC, 112–113
    family council meetings, 109
    formal recruitment sessions, 106–108
    incentives in recruitment for research
        projects, 121–122
    informal recruitment sessions, 109–110
    organizational structure of
        administration in CCRC, 104
    phone calls regarding new activities, 105
    process, 40–41
    in research settings, special
        considerations for, 110–112
    sessions, 106–110
    special considerations for recruiting in
        research settings, 110–112
Remote patient monitoring, 155
Research, 110
    research projects, incentives in
        recruitment and retention for,
        121–122
    research settings, recruiting in, 110–112
Residential communities for older adults,
    11–12
Residents, 120–121
Retention, 113
    activity director, 120–121
    building rapport, 115–116
    class time, 116–119
    incentives in retention for research
        projects, 121–122
    needs, 114–115
    office hours, 119–120
Robotics, 164–165

S

Search engine, 83
Second-level digital divide, 84
Self-efficacy, 88–90
Self-esteem, 88–89
Skype, 146
Social barriers, 97
Social isolation, 95
Social networks, 115
    social networking sites, 67
Spatial barriers, 97
"Starting with the basics" training
        program, 108
Stereotypical "tech person", 133
Stress of transition, 22
    adjusting to transition, 23–25
    feelings, 22–23
    impacts on social interactions and
        relationships, 25–26

T

Technology developments, 149
Technology training, 83–84, 141
    activity director in recruitment and
        retention, 120–121
    aging population demographics, 2–8
    attitudes toward ICTs, 85–88
    changing attitudes, 84
    incentives in recruitment and retention
        for research projects, 121–122
    for older adults in CCRCs, 1–2
    programs, 103
    quality of life outcomes, 94–99
    recruitment, 103–113
    residential communities for, 11–12
    retention, 113–120
    self-efficacy, 88–90
    technology classes, 84–85
    technology usage, 9–11, 91–93
    tech training, 99–100
    value of technology for, 9
Teleconferencing, healthcare via, 154–155
Telehealth, *see* Healthcare—delivery
Telemedicine, *see* Health—education
Telepresence, 164–165
Trainers, 132
    and assistants, 134–135
Training
    duration, 130–131
    location, 131

program, 125, 145
training personnel and methods,
consistency in, 135
Training decisions
anticipated numbers, 127–129
background and knowledge, 132
consistency in training personnel and
methods, 135
external contractor decisions, 136–139
factors and characteristics, 135–136
fit with CCRC population, 140
individual *vs.* group training sessions,
129–130
interpersonal characteristics, 132–134
number of trainers and assistants
needed, 134–135
training duration, 130–131
training location, 131
troubleshoot, 131
uniqueness of specific CCRC
populations, 125–127
Twitter, 68

U

Uniqueness of specific CCRC populations,
125–127

University of Maryland, Baltimore County
(UMBC), 33
U.S. trends, 6–9

V

Videoconferencing, healthcare via,
154–155
Virtual healthcare, 154
healthcare via teleconferencing
or videoconferencing,
154–155
mobile health applications,
155–157
Visual ability, 58–59
Volunteers, 139

W

Windows Vista to Windows 8, 160–163
Wiring, 42

Y

YouTube, 67